Color Atlas of

Peripheral Vascular Diseases

William F Walker
DSc, Ch.M, FRCS, FRCS (Edin.), FRS (Edin.)

Consultant Surgeon
Ninewells Hospital,
Dundee and Reader in Surgery
at University of Dundee,
Scotland

Year Book Medical Publishers, Inc
35 East Wacker Drive, Chicago

Series Editor: G. Barry Carruthers, MD(London)
ISBN 0-8151-9083-2
Library of Congress Catalog Card Number: 80-81016

Distributed in Continental North, South and Central America,
Hawaii, Puerto Rico and the Philippines by
Year Book Medical Publishers, Inc.
By arrangement with Wolfe Medical Publications Ltd.
Printed by Smeets-Weert, Holland

Other books in this series already published:
Color Atlas of General Pathology
Color Atlas of Oro-Facial Diseases
Color Atlas of Ophthalmological Diagnosis
Color Atlas of Renal Diseases
Color Atlas of Venereology
Color Atlas of Dermatology
Color Atlas of Infectious Diseases
Color Atlas of Ear, Nose & Throat Diagnosis
Color Atlas of Rheumatology
Color Atlas of Microbiology
Color Atlas of Forensic Pathology
Color Atlas of Pediatrics
Color Atlas of Histology
Color Atlas of General Surgical Diagnosis
Color Atlas of Physical Signs in General Medicine
Color Atlas of Tropical Medicine & Parasitology
Color Atlas of Human Anatomy
Color Atlas of Cardiac Pathology
Color Atlas of Histological Staining Techniques
Atlas of Cardiology: ECGs and Chest X-Rays
Color Atlas of Neuropathology
Color Atlas of Oral Medicine
Color Atlas of Oral Anatomy
Color Atlas of Periodontology
Color Atlas of Gynecological Surgery
(Volumes 1–4; Volumes 5 and 6 in preparation)
Color Atlas of Liver Disease
Color Atlas of Pedodontics
Color Atlas of Endocrinology
Color Atlas of Ocular Tumors
Color Atlas of Pathogenic Fungi
Color Atlas of Temporal Bone Surgical Anatomy
Color Atlas of Tumor Histopathology
Color Atlas of Diabetes

Contents

Introduction

Vascular disease in its various forms accounts for nearly half the deaths in the western world and for a considerable loss of work and suffering.

Fortunately over the past 30 years there have been rapid developments in our understanding of vascular physiology, pathology, aetiology and therefore to some extent its prevention, clinical presentation and finally treatment. Because the last is continually evolving and changing, only the principles will be discussed here. Particular attention is focused on visual recognition of the various states as these even in the early stage may be diagnostic.

Vascular disease is not necessarily a disease of one area of the vascular system but is usually widespread with emphasis in a localised area. It is necessary therefore to consider the whole patient since coexistent disease, the presence of diabetes or hyperlipidaemia, or other conditions such as cancer have a considerable effect on prognosis and treatment.

This book presents vascular disease in a pictorial form. It should be a useful supplement to the many detailed and excellent books on vascular surgery.

Acknowledgements

It is a pleasure to record my indebtedness to my colleagues and friends in vascular surgery, in particular to my old chief, Sir Donald Douglas, who introduced me to vascular surgery and taught me the rudiments. This atlas owes much to the generous help of friends and colleagues including:

Mr P H Dickinson

Dr G F A Howie

Dr P B James

Prof. K G Lowe

Dr Pathi

Dr D G Rushton

Dr J W Shaw

Mr D W Short

Mr M G Walker

Dr M Wilkinson

Mr R A B Wood

My thanks are also due to the publishers for their forbearance, guidance and help. Finally, the proof was read by Mr A D Irvine to whom I am indebted.

1 Diseases of the arteries

1

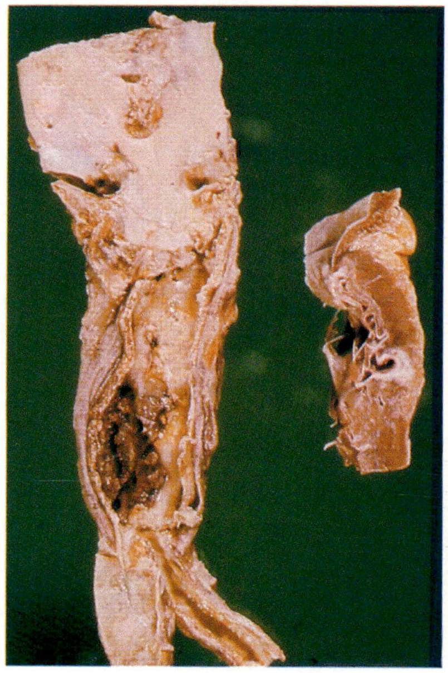

1 **Arteriosclerosis obliterans** (ASO) is the commonest arterial disease. Subintimal deposition of atheroma produces narrowing of the vessels and superimposed ulceration of the atheromatous nodule results in thrombus formation. Severe disease in the aorta and common iliac arteries is present with ulceration and thrombosis. On the right narrowing of the coronary artery and myocardial ischaemic fibrosis is visible.

2

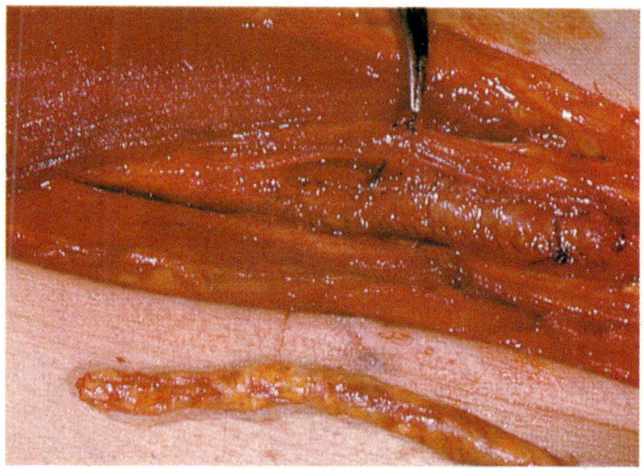

2 **Atheroma** refers to the 'porridge-like' deposit below the intima. In this case it has become organised and extended up and down the artery for some distance forming a plug or roll. The whole plug can be excised (endarterectomy) and the defect in the artery filled by a patch of vein (patch angioplasty), as shown here.

3

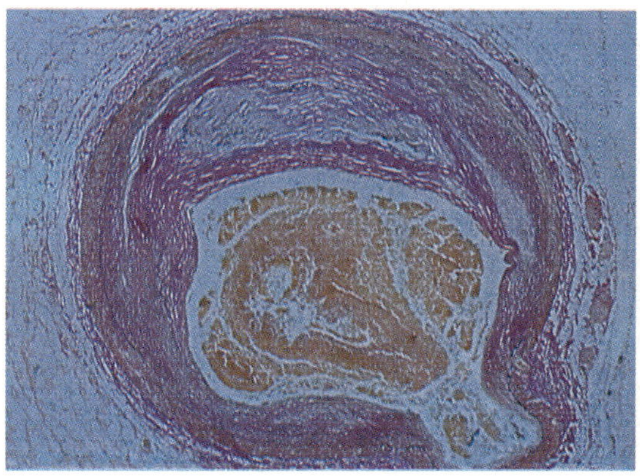

3 **Subintimal atheroma.** This histological section shows the narrowing of the artery with subintimal atheroma. The atheromatous plaque shows as a blue-red area in the top of the picture.

4

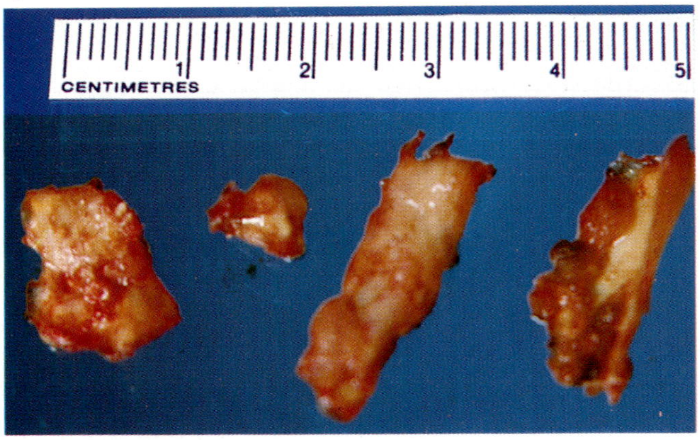

4 Atheroma in common iliac artery. Atheromatous material excised from the common iliac artery of a patient at operation. It illustrates the various stages from yellow patches on the left specimen through ulceration to old and recent thrombus.

5

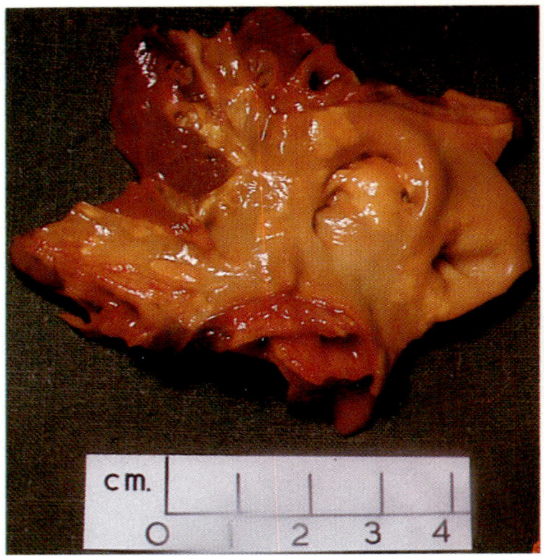

5 Mitral stenosis atheroma. Atheroma may even involve the pulmonary artery secondary, as here, to pulmonary hypertension due to mitral stenosis. The lipoid material is shown as yellow plaques and represents the earliest form of the disease.

Acute ischaemia

Occlusion of the arterial lumen may be due to a number of causes which may be localised or related to a general condition.

Local	**General**
Thrombosis	Poor blood flow e.g. shock heart failure
Embolism	Blood dyscrasia e.g. polycythaemia leukaemia thrombocythaemia cold agglutinins
Tourniquet	
Splint	
Vasospasm	
Cold injury	
Injury e.g. trauma, operation or infection	
Ergot	

The clinical features of acute ischaemia are pain, pallor, pulselessness, paralysis and paraesthesia going on to sensory loss.

6

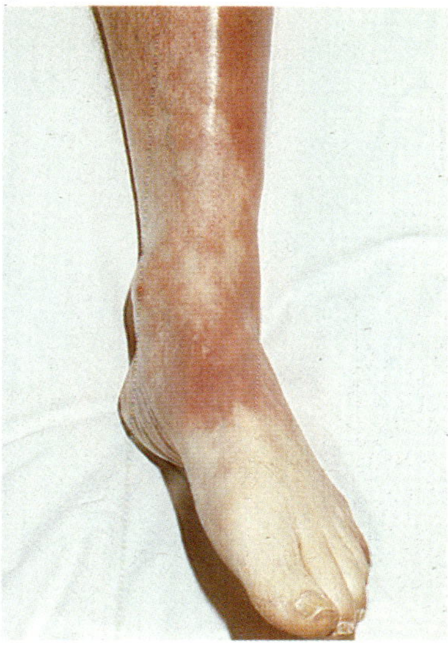

7

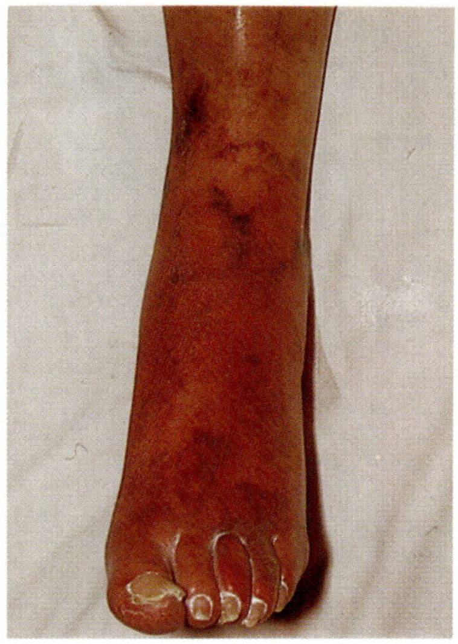

6 Acute ischaemia: early change. The early change is shown in this leg. The main artery was clamped during resection of an aortic aneurysm. The foot shows the waxy pallor of bloodlessness and above is the reactive hyperaemia of recovering flow.

7 Acute ischaemia: later change. The later changes of acute ischaemia are shown, a blotchy cyanosis widespread and coalescing with extravasation of blood into blisters. This goes on to frank gangrene. In this case the cause was an embolus from the left atrium.

8

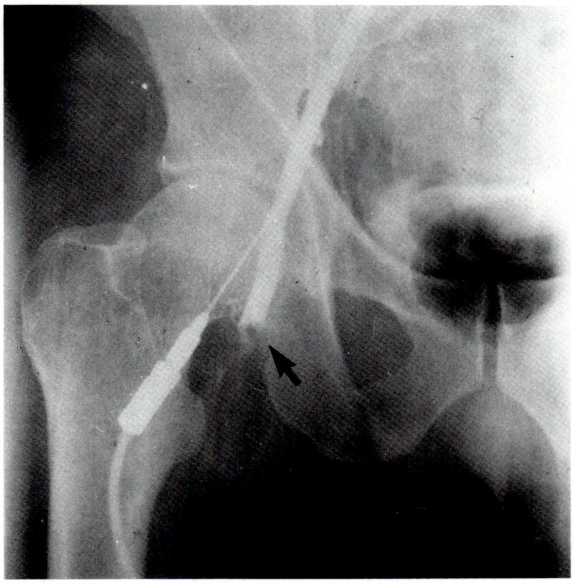

8 Embolus in right femoral artery. The arteriogram shows an embolus, recognised by the crescentic appearance at the lower part of the contrast material, in the left femoral artery. Usually with an embolus there is no previous history of claudication and a possible primary source, for example cardiac infarct, atrial fibrillation, or mitral valve disease is evident.

9

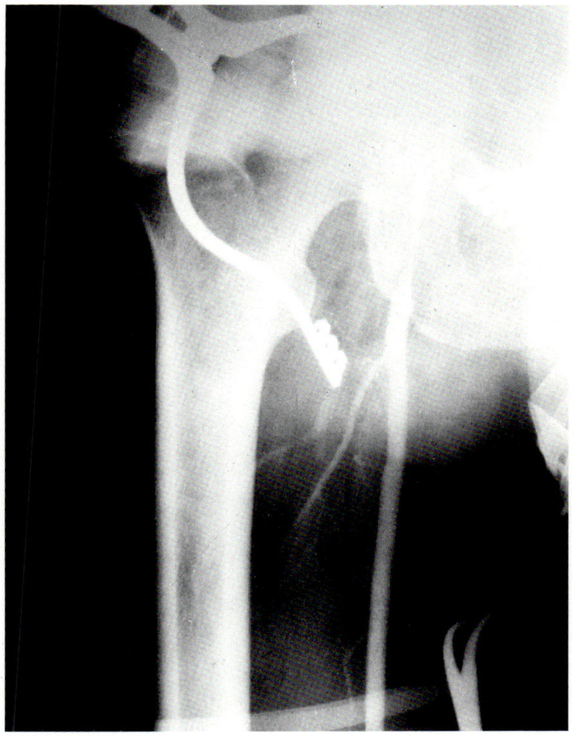

9 **The operative arteriogram** in the previous case was taken immediately after removal of the embolus under local anaesthetic.

10

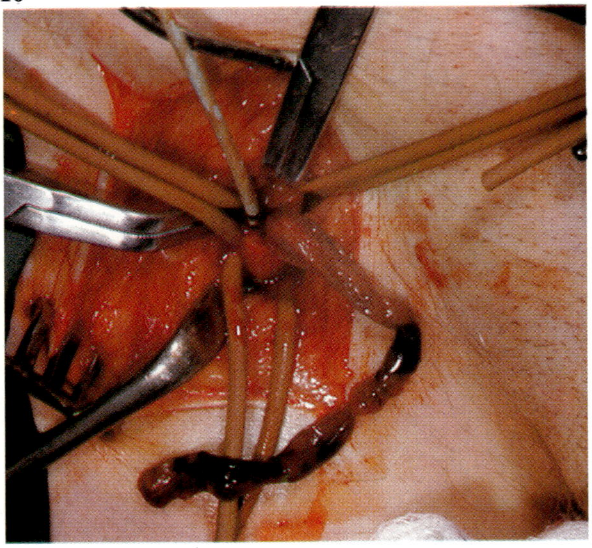

10 Embolus in right femoral artery. An embolus is being removed from the right femoral artery by a Fogarty catheter. Old clot it just visible with relatively new clot at the upper end. In embolectomy the catheter slips easily up the artery. If removal is difficult this usually means extensive underlying ASO and most likely a thrombosis rather than embolus. The ultimate prognosis for limb survival with thrombosis is not so good.

11

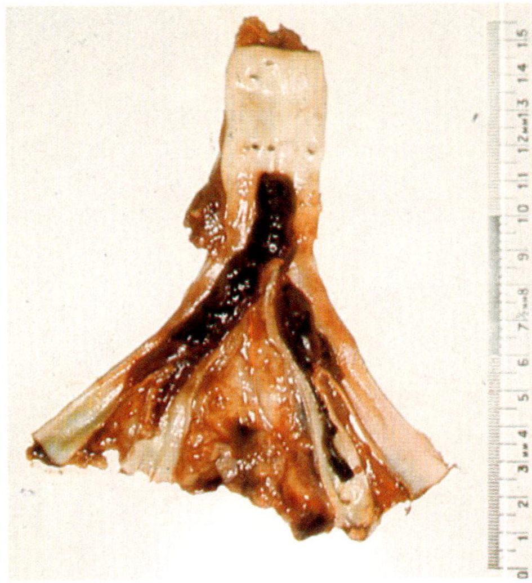

11 Embolus at aortic bifurcation. The classical first site of lodgement of an embolus at the aortic bifurcation. The patient had sudden onset of pain and pallor in both lower limbs with absence of the femoral pulses.

12

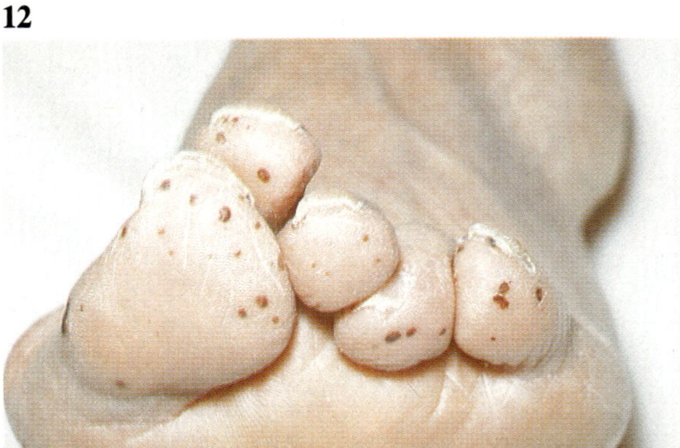

12 Microemboli in toes. Embolisation need not necessarily lead to massive ischaemia. In this case microemboli are seen in the toes, which were otherwise warm and normal in colour. with apparently good venous filling.

13

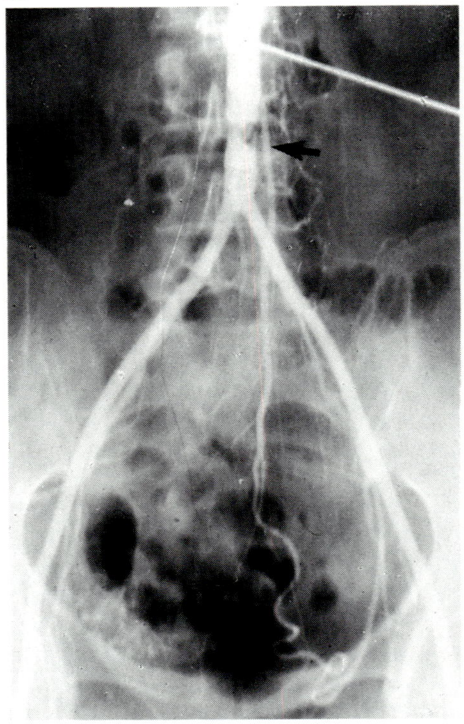

13 Aortic thrombus. The aortogram showed the most likely source of emboli in the above patient—an aortic thrombus. This was removed at operation and no more emboli were seen.

14

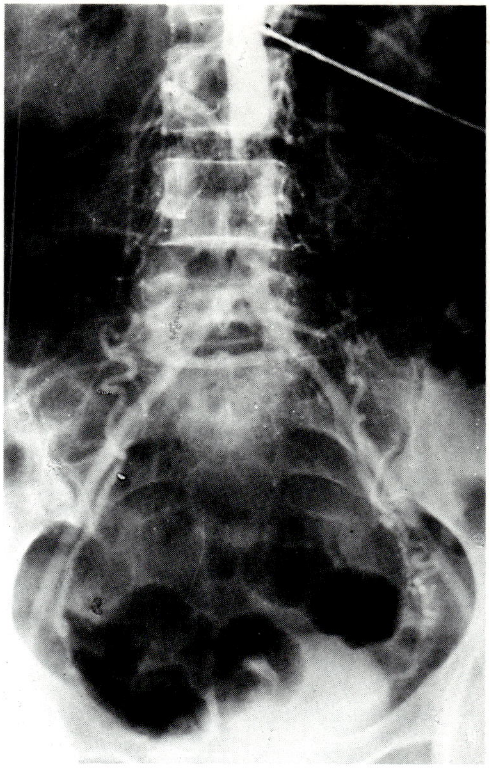

14 Peripheral embolisation. In another patient with peripheral embolisation the aortic thrombosis and atheromatous disease was much greater. Indeed almost complete obliteration has occurred.

15

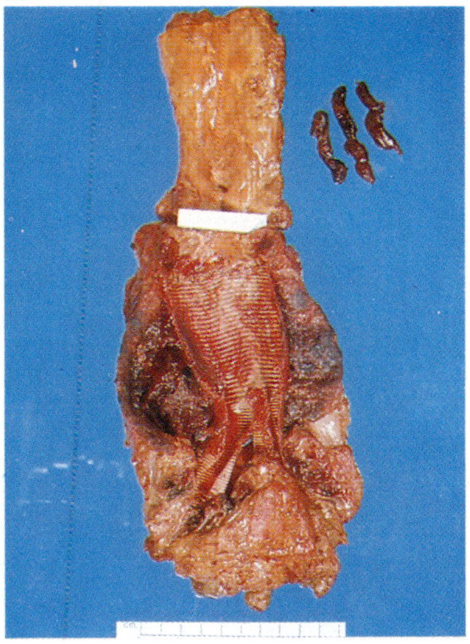

15 Distal ischaemia. Occasionally emboli may arise from an aortic trouser-graft prosthesis. This prosthesis was inserted for a leaking aortic aneurysm. The patient developed distal ischaemia in the right leg. The source was thrombus in the right limb of the graft at the site of the anastomosis. Despite removal of the proximal clots the patient died. The upper aorta shows the yellow streaking of atheroma.

16

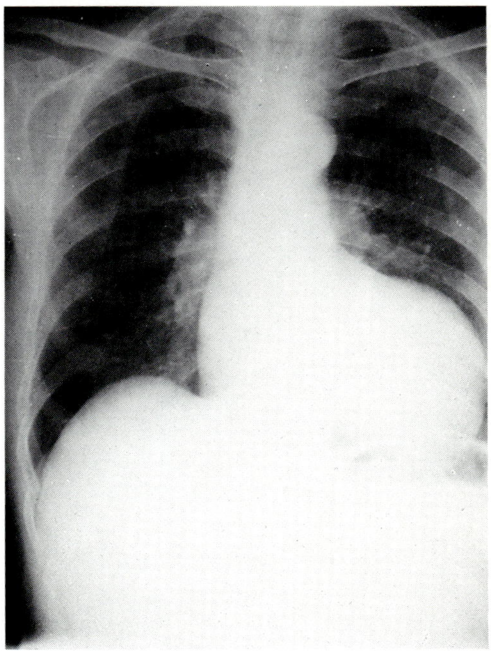

16 Aneurysm of left ventricle. One of the rare sources of embolus is shown—an aneurysm of left ventricle. The patient had a major infarct some months previously.

17

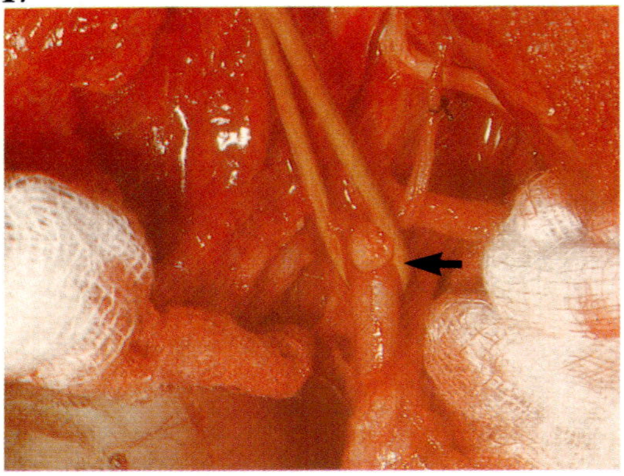

17 Embolus in lower aorta. A very rare type of embolus lodged in lower aorta—a portion of an atrial myxoma. The diagnosis is based on the peculiar type of material seen on opening up the artery or brought down by the Fogarty catheter. The material is extruding in front of the retractor.

18

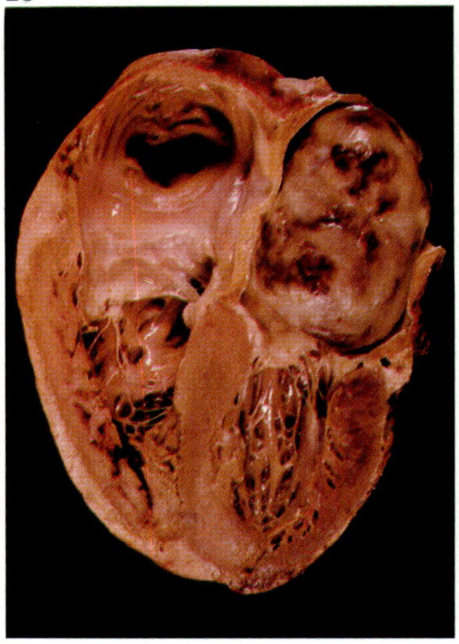

18 Myxoma of left atrium. A large tumour can be seen filling the left atrium. On section it was found to be a myxoma. Death in this case was due to obstruction of the mitral valve with cardiac failure.

19

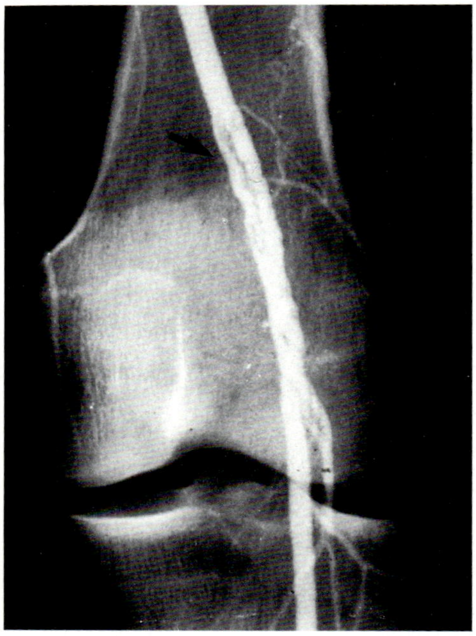

19 Thrombus in popliteal artery. Acute ischaemia may be due to thrombosis usually occurring in an artery diseased with atheroma. The arteriogram shows thrombus in the popliteal artery. The patient had ishcaemic changes mostly affecting the right big toe but the whole foot was pale and cold. Removal of the clot by Fogarty catheter improved the condition, although the underlying atheroma remained.

20

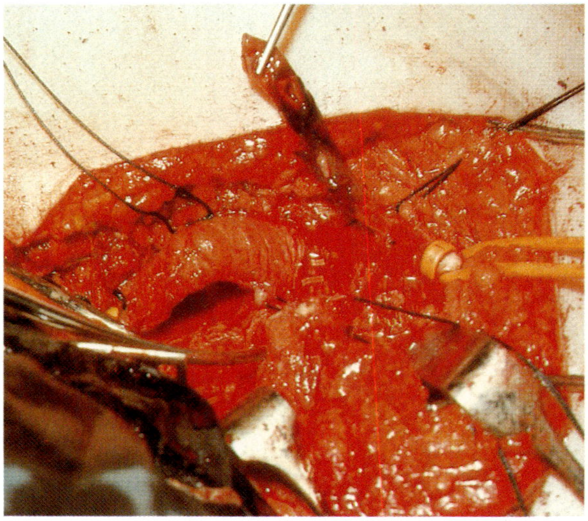

20 Partial obstruction of artery. Where an artery is kinked over a partial obstruction, in this case a cervical rib, thrombosis may occur. The thrombus is shown being removed at open operation. A portion of the thrombus could easily separate as an embolus.

21

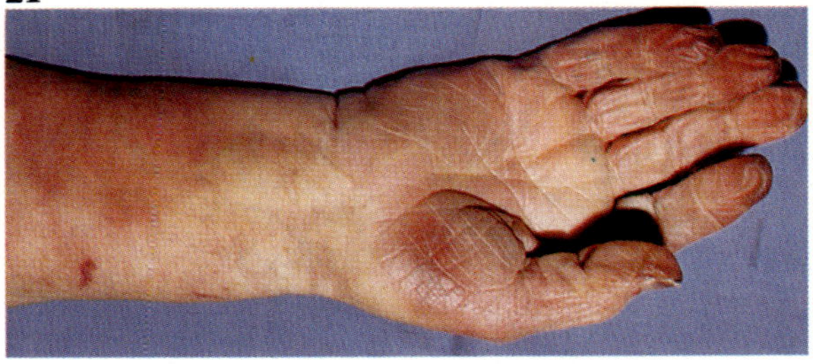

21 Axillary artery thrombosis. Acute on chronic ischaemia is suggested by the mottled cyanosis, and blistering with obvious loss of tissue turgor shows in the shrivelled finger tips. This resulted from an axillary artery thrombosis.

22

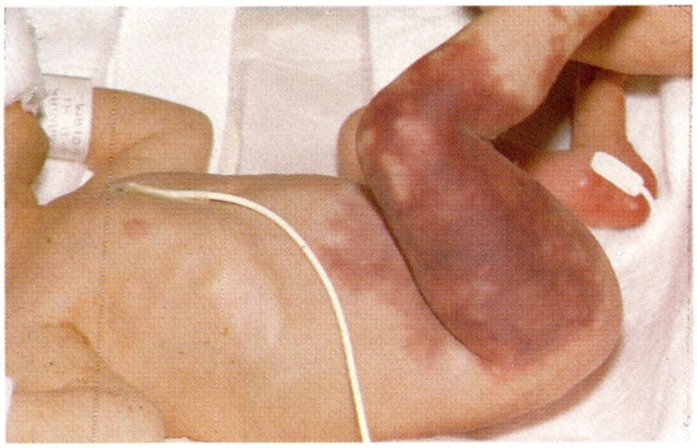

22 Acute ischaemic change in the skin of a baby who had injection of a toxic substance into the umbilical artery.

23

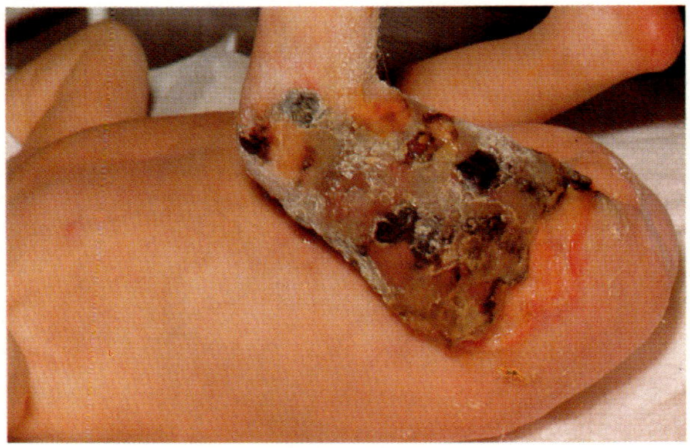

23 Skin graft. The skin in the above case became gangrenous and sloughed off. Subsequent grafting of skin produced a satisfactory result, with survival of the child.

24

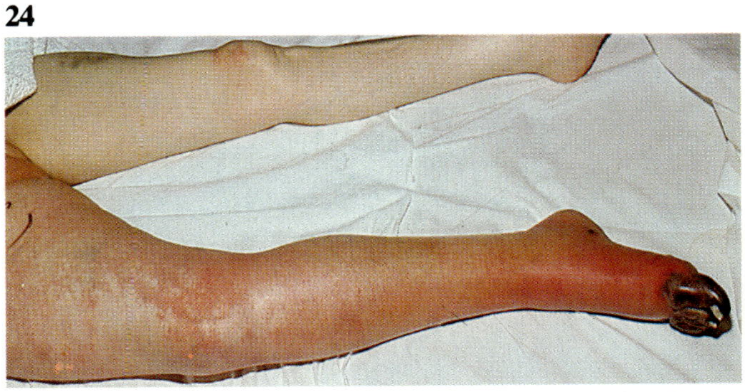

24 Phlegmasia caerulea dolens. Acute ischaemia may have an underlying venous cause as in phlegmasia caerulea dolens where back pressure and limb swelling, with or without possible secondary thrombosis, may produce marked ischaemia which may lead to gangrene. The gross swelling, cyanotic appearance and moist gangrene suggest a primary venous problem. Venous thrombectomy was done to relieve the pressure and the cyanosis diminished.

Acute ischaemia may go on to gangrene.

2 Gangrene

25

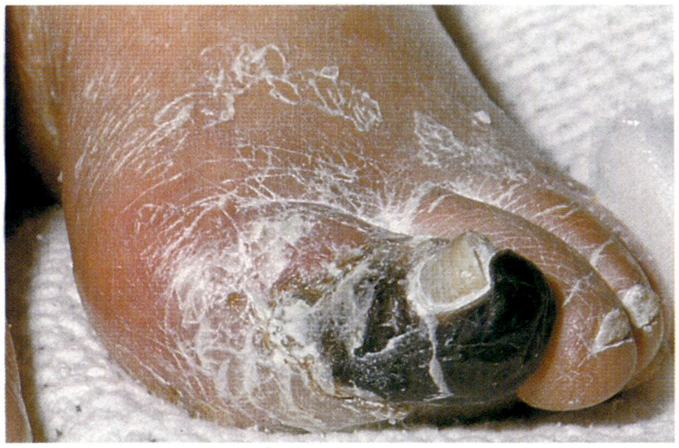

25 Typical dry gangrene due to diffuse ASO blocking the femoral artery and affecting also the vessels below the knee. This patient had a history of claudication in the calf muscles and pain in the big toe and second toe.

26

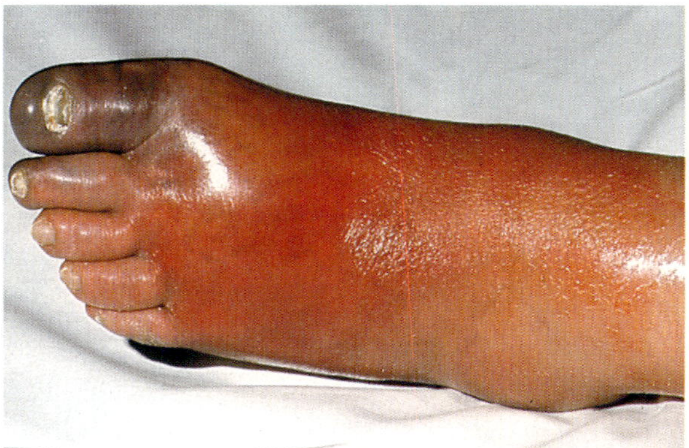

26 Moist gangrene. This is a case of moist gangrene caused by deep vein thrombosis. The gross swelling of the leg and the blister formation are typical.

27

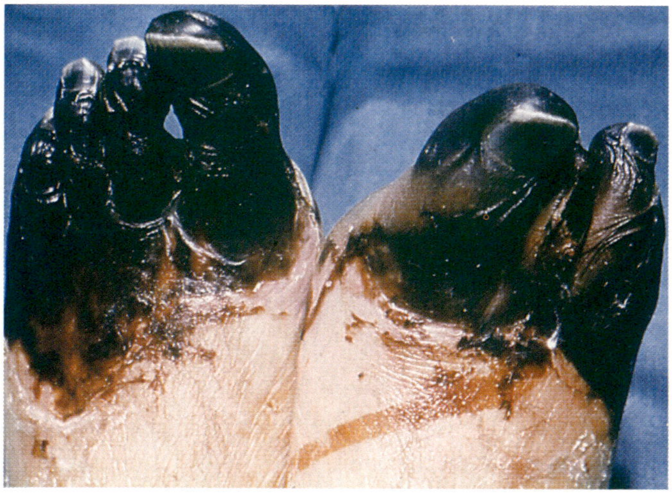

27 Another form of moist gangrene at a later stage when some mummification has taken place. This patient had a cancer of the pancreas—a relationship which is well described, interesting, but difficult to elucidate.

28

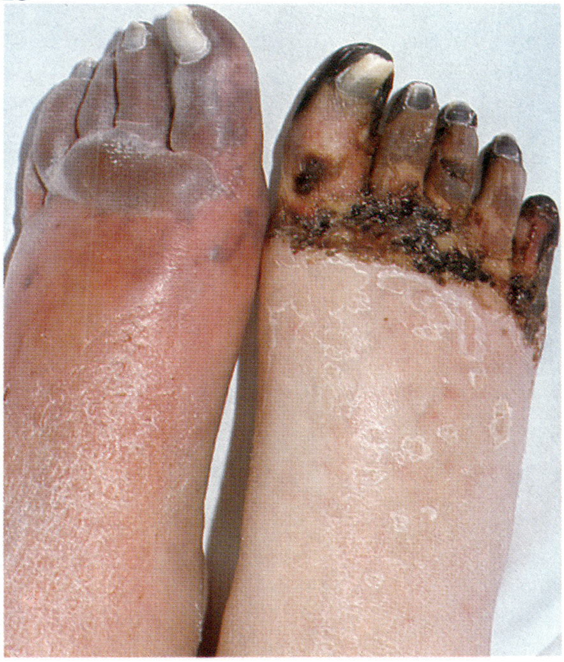

28 Dry and moist gangrene. A rather unusual combination of dry gangrene in the right foot and moist in the left. The dry gangrene was due to ASO: the moist was due to a superadded deep venous thrombosis (DVT) in the left leg.

29

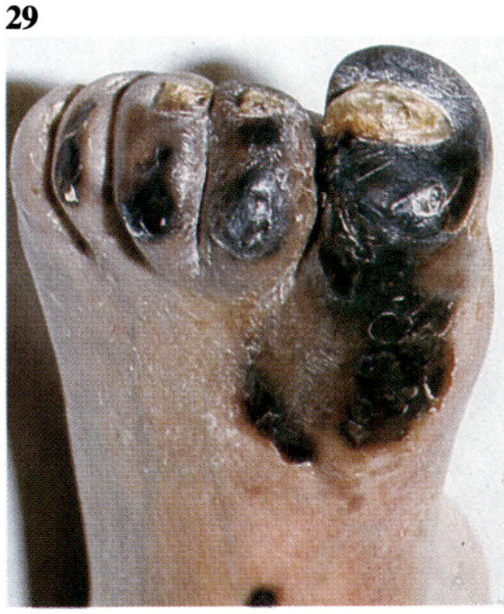

29 Diabetic gangrene is likely to combine the dry and moist forms. The latter was due to superadded infection.

30

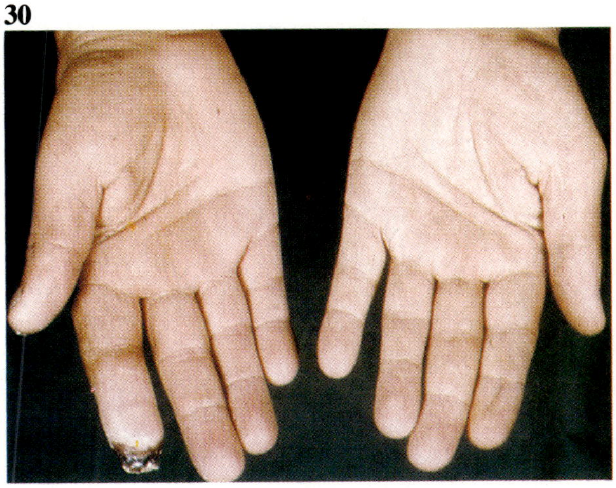

30 Raynaud's disease with gangrene of the tip of the right forefinger, initially due to spasm and then due to digital artery thrombosis.

31

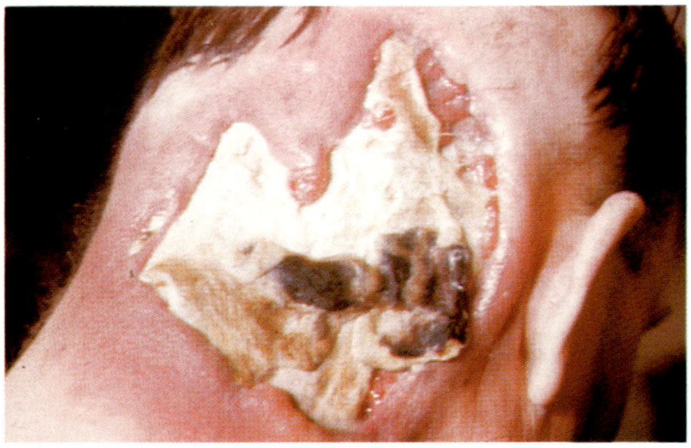

31 Another form of diabetic gangrene occurs in a carbuncle in a diabetic. The central skin becomes ischaemic due to pressure and a cutting off of the blood supply with sloughing of the skin.

32

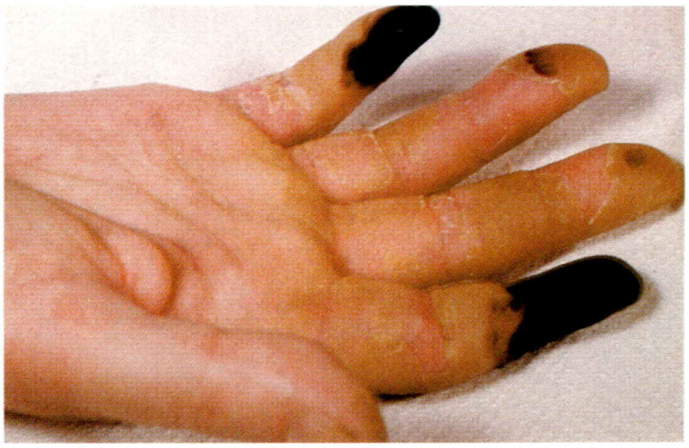

32 Digital gangrene. A cervical rib can result in gangrene of the digits due to emboli showering off from a thrombus in the distorted subclavian artery, with possibly an aneurysm formed.

33

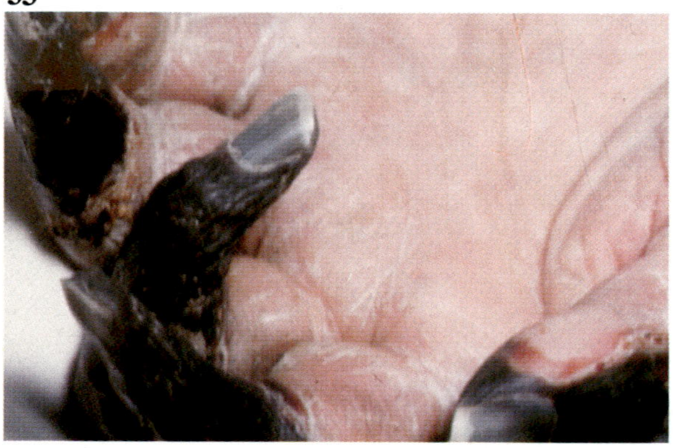

33 Gangrene from thrombosis of axillary artery. This resulted from thrombosis of the axillary artery due to ASO. A portion of the thrombus had embolised down to plug the radial and ulnar arteries.

34

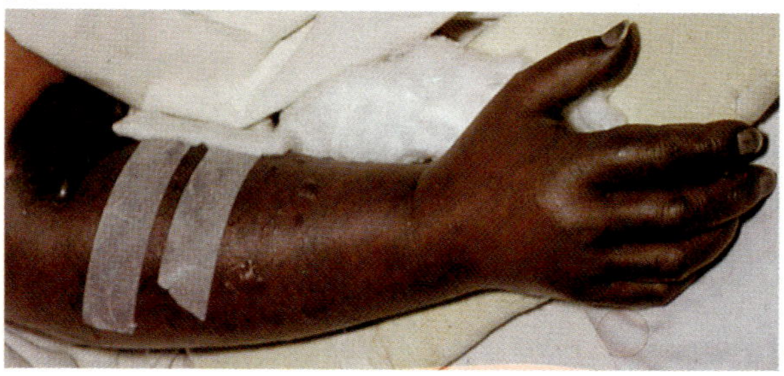

34 Gangrene from thrombosis of the axillary vein is rather rare. The deep blue discolouration and the blebs of venous obstruction are present.

35

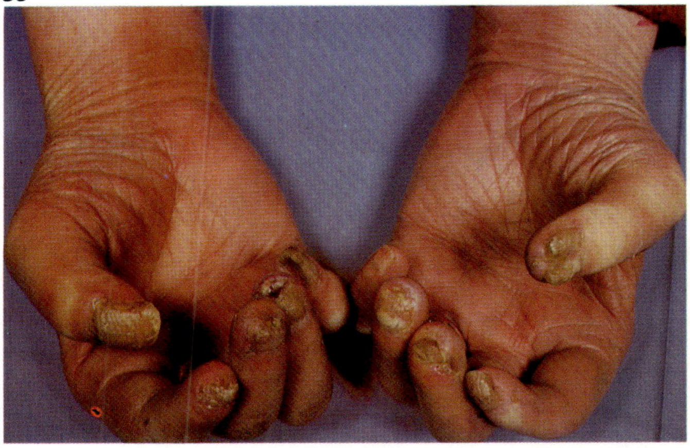

35 Gangrene due to scleroderma. In scleroderma the changes in the small vessels of the hand are such as to produce blockage with gangrene and ulceration of the tips of the fingers.

36

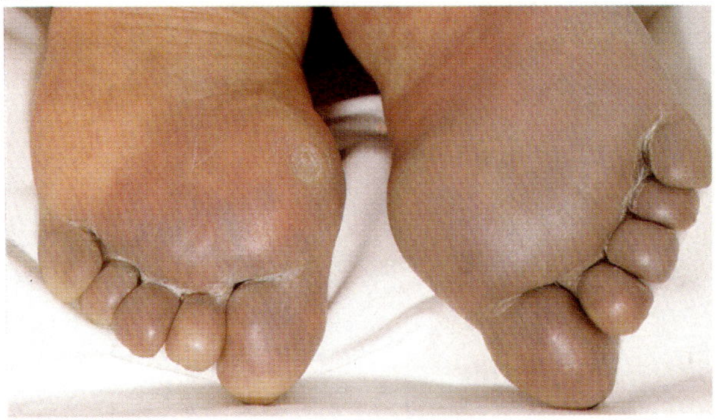

36 Distal gangrene. Intravascular coagulation associated with shock may produce a distal form of gangrene as in this patient.

37

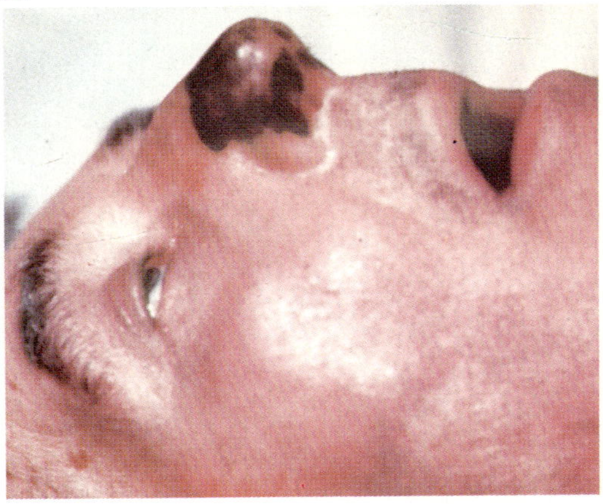

37 Coronary thrombosis. Low output failure in this patient was due to a massive coronary thrombosis. Usually severe ischaemic changes are noted in the ears, fingers and sometimes the nose. Actual gangrene of the tip of the nose is rare.

38

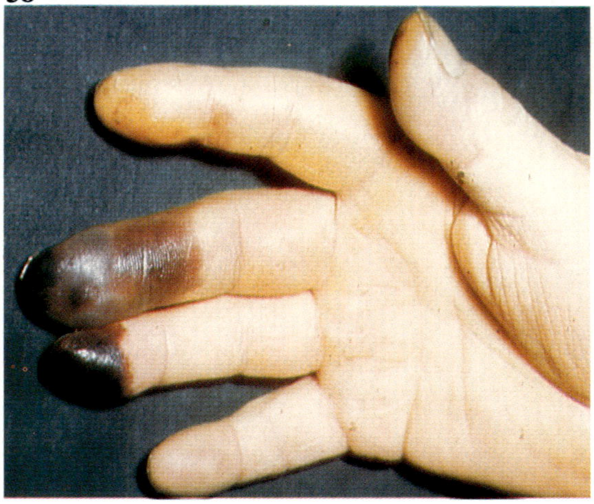

38 Gangrene due to trauma to digital vessels. An interesting case where a man was bitten by an insane person in two fingers of the hand. He developed septicaemia shock, peripheral circulatory failure, and gangrene in the fingers presumably due to previous trauma to the digital vessels.

39

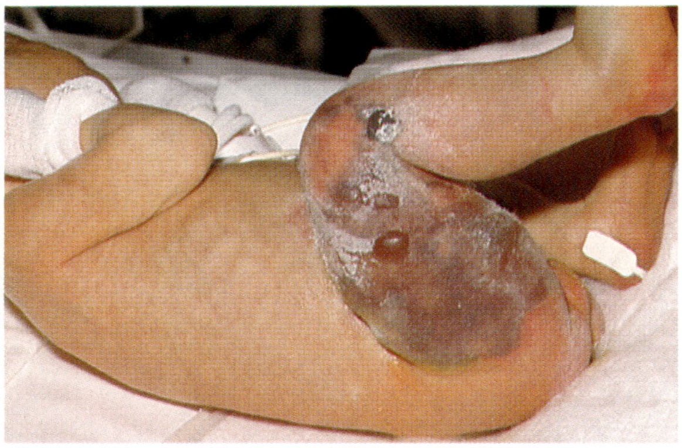

39 Gangrene due to intravascular injection may, as in this child, produce gangrene of a limited extent.

40

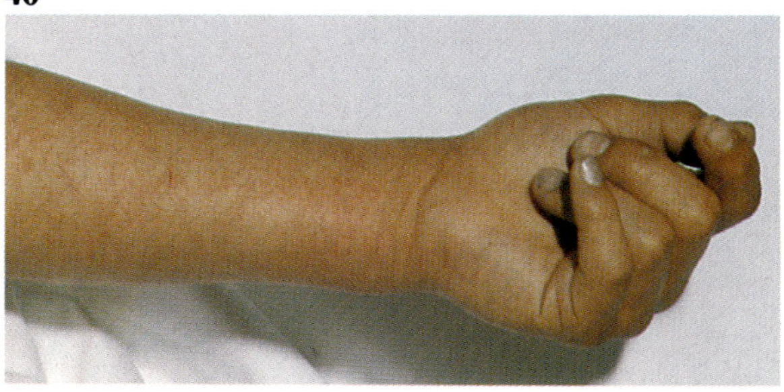

40 Intra-arterial injection in a drug addict is perhaps becoming a little more common than in the past. The irritant fluid produces arterial thrombosis. The fingernails of the fourth and fifth fingers are cyanosed.

41

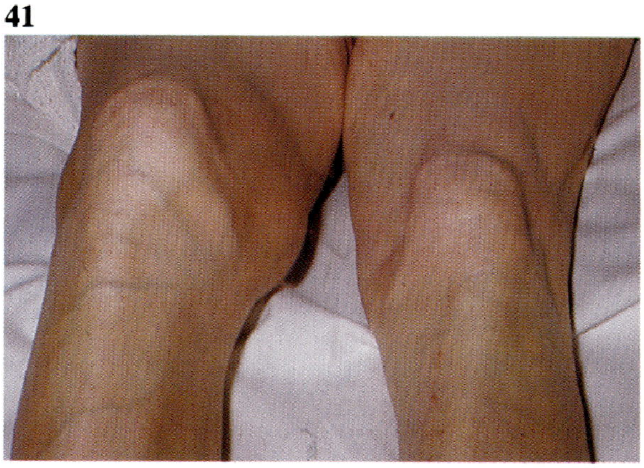

41 Thrombosis in a popliteal aneurysm is often followed by gangrene of the foot. The aneurysm in the right popliteal artery can be seen on the medial side of the knee.

42

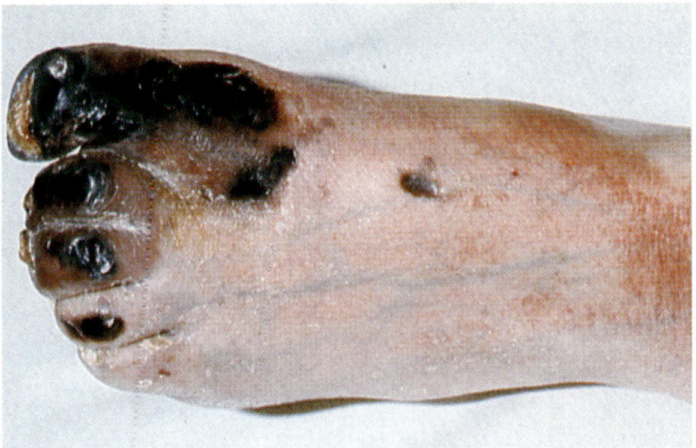

42 Gangrene resulting from popliteal thrombosis. This patient needed a below-the-knee amputation.

43

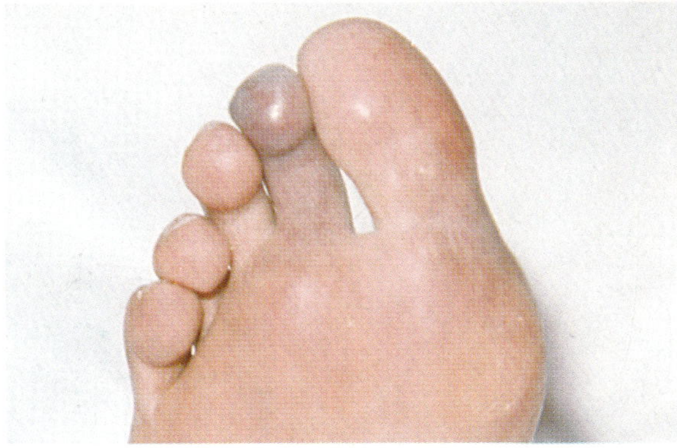

43 Polycythaemia. This patient presented with gangrene of the second toe on the right foot. The foot pulses were normal. Blood examination revealed a marked degree of polycythaemia.

44

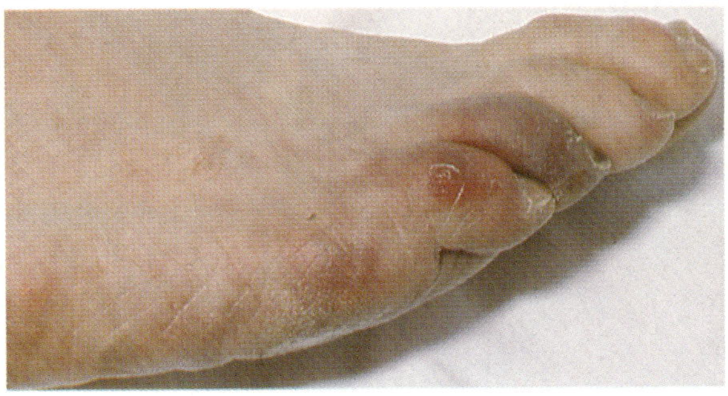

44 Frostbite gangrene. Frostbite was considered a cause of gangrene in this patient; he was found out in the snow and his foot pulses were present. In frostbite there is actual freezing of the tissues by dry cold.

45

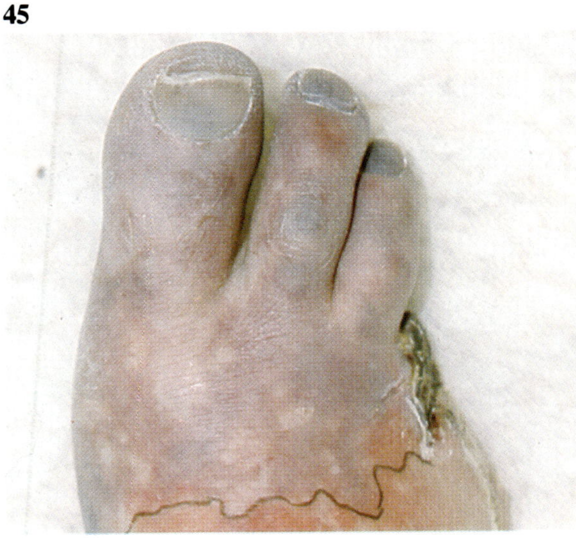

45 Digital gangrene. The lateral toes were removed because of pain and the others became gangrenous. Digital gangrene with good foot pulses strongly suggests embolism from proximal atheromatous disease with ulceration and thrombosis.

46

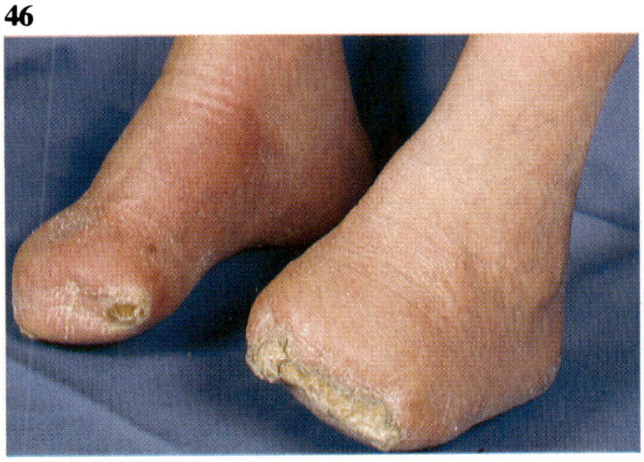

46 **Trench foot** is the result of prolonged exposure of the feet to a cold wet environment above freezing point. This patient was a soldier in World War I. He had to undergo amputations for gangrene.

47

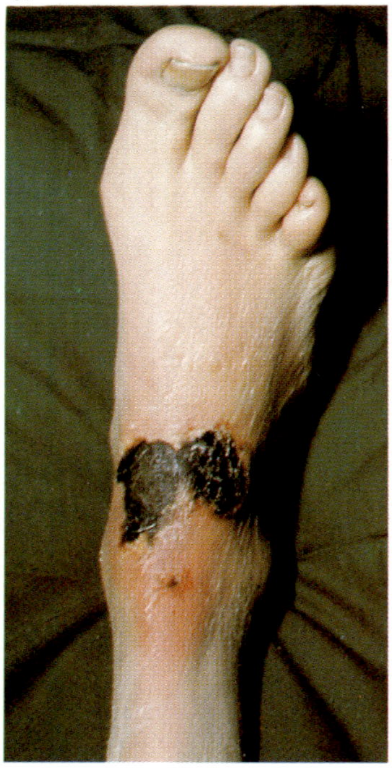

48

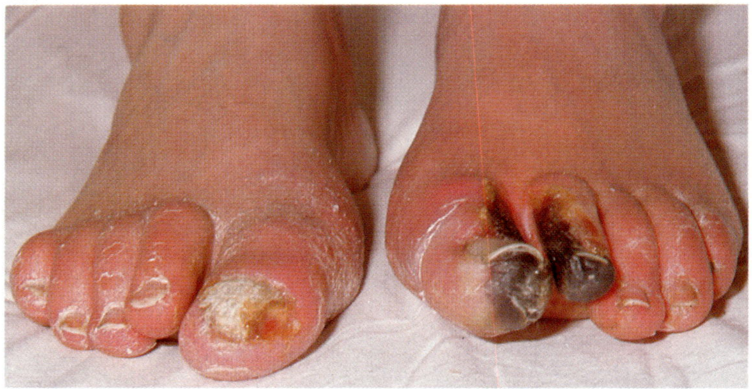

48 Buerger's disease, which affects mainly the distal lower limb vessels, may be accompanied by gangrene as in this 42-year-old man. He smoked 60 cigarettes per day.

47 Skin gangrene. Pressure by excessively tight bandages can produce gangrene of the skin.

49

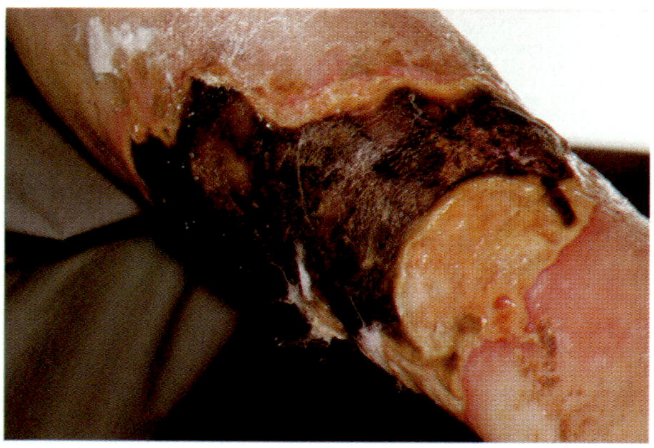

49 Gangrene with extensive sloughing can occur after too extensive undermining of the skin in an operation for varicose veins.

50

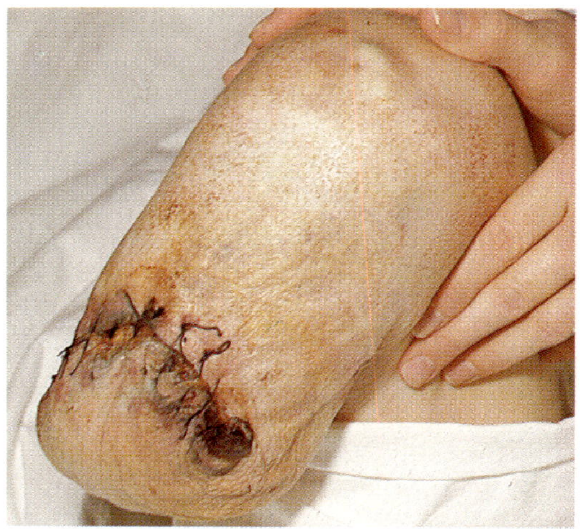

50 Tension gangrene. An example of tension gangrene where the vascular supply, which is usually precarious to begin with, becomes obliterated by tension in the wound.

51

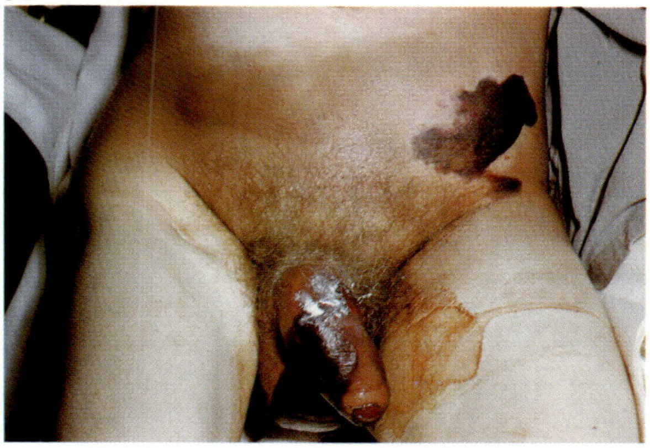

51 In Fournier's gangrene there is both tension in grossly swollen tissue and intravascular thrombosis from surrounding sepsis.

52

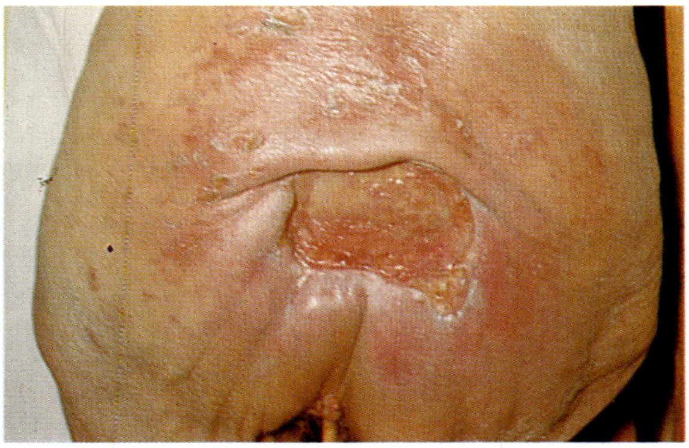

52 Bed sore. Obliteration of blood supply by direct pressure produces the typical bed sore.

53

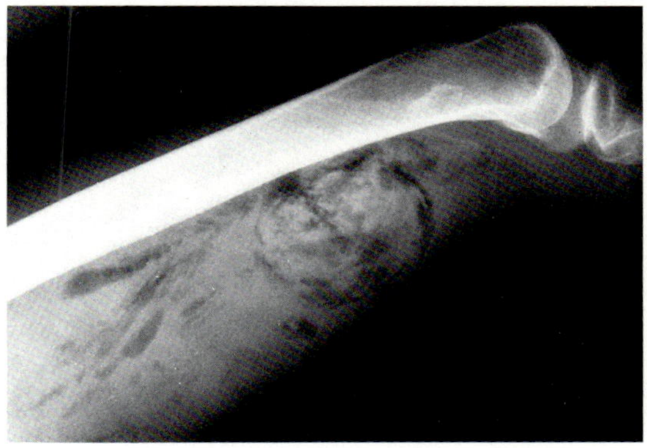

53 Gas gangrene due to clostridial infection. The combination of organismal gas production and muscle necrosis produces marked swelling with impairment of circulation. The gas can be seen in the x-ray of the leg.

54

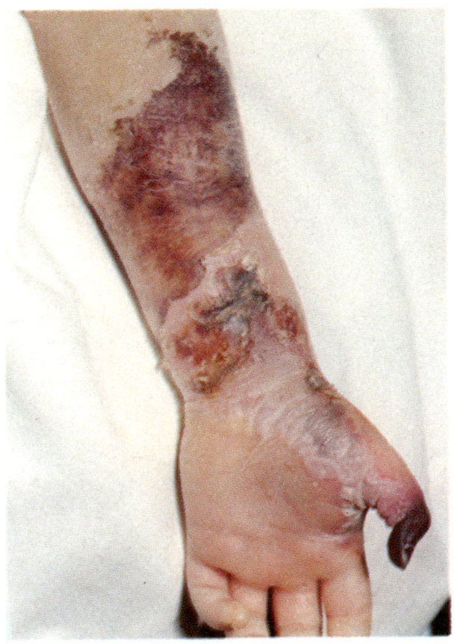

54 Pressure gangrene may be caused by tight plasters or splints. This case shows result of too tight a split in treatment of a fracture of either radius or ulna.

3 Chronic arterial occlusive disease

55

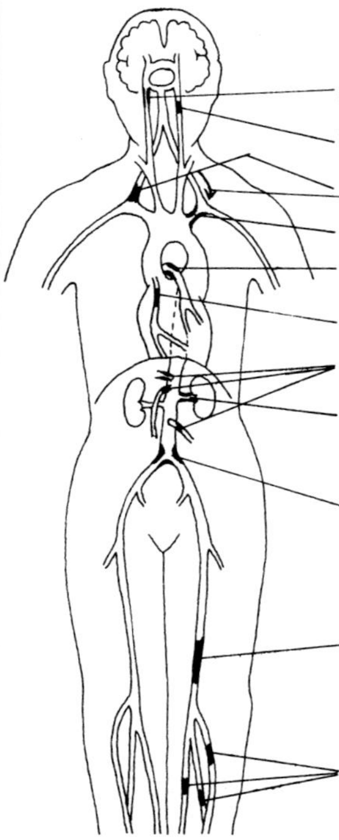

Condition	Symptoms	Arteries
stenosis	little stroke syndrome	internal
block	major stroke	carotid
stenosis or block	giddiness	vertebral
stenosis or block	subclavian steal syndrome ischaemia of arm or hand	subclavian
stenosis	angina pectoris	coronaries
block	coronary thrombosis	
stenosis or block	abdominal angina	coeliac superior } mesenteric inferior
stenosis	hypertension	renal
stenosis or block	Leriche syndrome (intermittent claudication of buttocks)	aorta
block	intermittent claudication of calf muscles	femoral
block	gangrene of foot	below knee arteries and femoral

55 **Although arteriosclerosis obliterans (ASO)** is a generalised disease it does have a predilection for certain sites. There may be complete occlusion or stenosis or narrowing and these are shown with the related syndromes.

Lower limb disease

The main site of occlusion in about 60 per cent of cases is in the superficial femoral artery with ischaemia of the tissues below the knee. Although the symptoms are usually unilateral the disease is often bilateral.

Clinical features

Clinical features depend on the efficiency of the collateral circulation. Two types of pain are experienced: *intermittent claudication*, where pain is felt in the calf or less commonly in the foot when a certain distance is walked, and *rest pain* where the discomfort is felt in the foot even at rest.

In the patient with claudication some pulses will be absent or much diminished and on auscultation a bruit may be heard. Where nutritional disturbance is present the affected limb will be colder than the other, possibly paler especially on elevation of the limb and there may be rubor on dependancy. Ischaemic changes may be apparent in the lower legs or feet with hair loss, smooth skin, unhealthy nails or frank necrotic changes.

As the disease is generalised a full examination of the cardiovascular system is necessary with exclusion also of anaemia, polycythaemia, diabetes and collagen disorders. Clinical myocardial ischaemic symptoms should be noted.

56

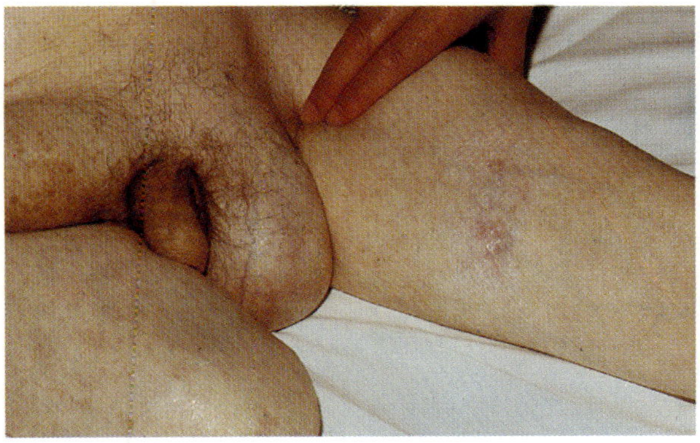

56 The femoral pulse is felt at the mid-inguinal point and is compared in volume with that on the other side. If it is diminished a thrill may be felt and a bruit heard. This would suggest proximal arterial narrowing.

57

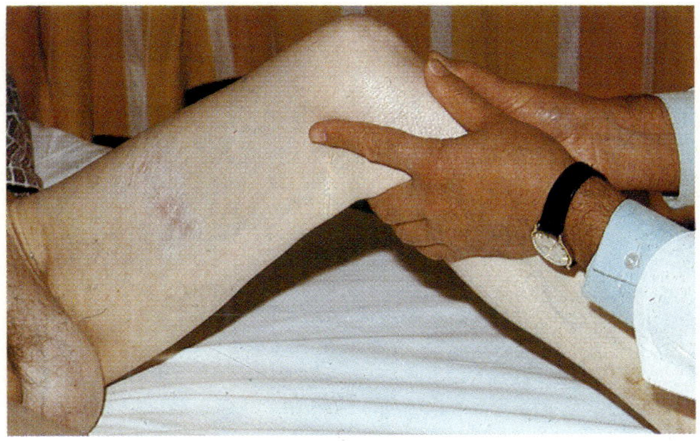

57 The popliteal pulse is most easily felt with the knee flexed either as shown, or with the patient supine and felt by direct pressure against the femur. In the obese and heavily muscled it may be difficult to feel this pulse even if present.

58

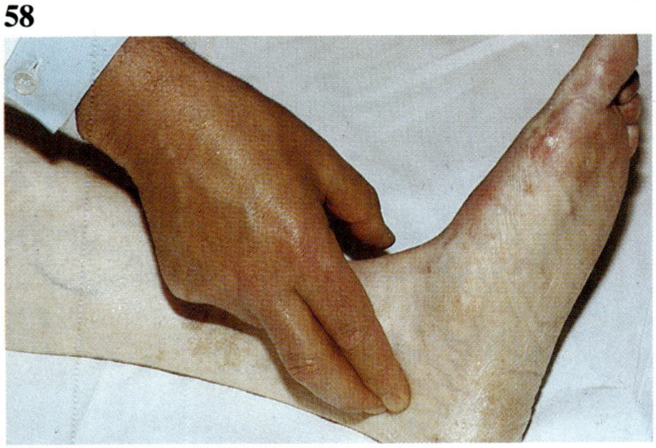

58 The posterior tibial pulse is usually easily felt in the groove behind the medial malleolus.

59

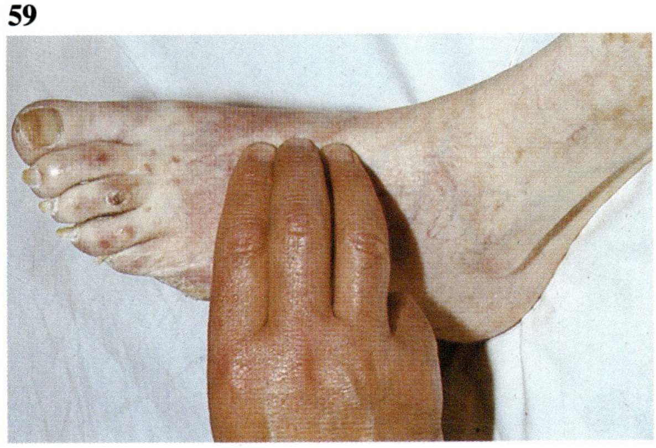

59 The dorsalis pedis pulse is felt just lateral to the extensor hallucis tendon, and just above the ankle in the same line is the anterior tibial pulse.

60

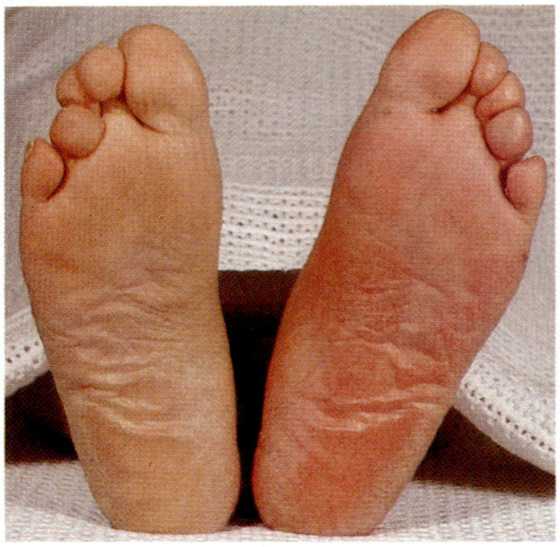

60 Intermittent claudication. The soles of the feet are observed with the patient lying flat. This patient had intermittent claudication of the right foot at distances of 100 metres. Both feet are well coloured but there is just the suspicion that the right foot is paler than the left.

61

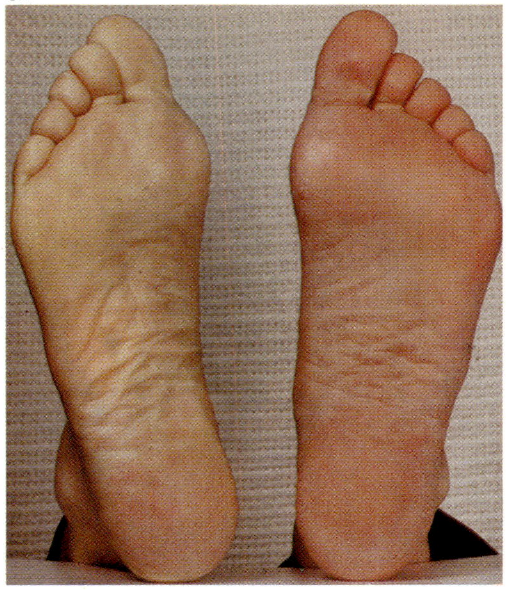

61 Ischaemia pallor. Elevation of the legs particularly with exercise may, if ischaemia is severe, produce pallor of the affected sole, because the blood has to be pumped up against gravity and venous emptying is increased.

62

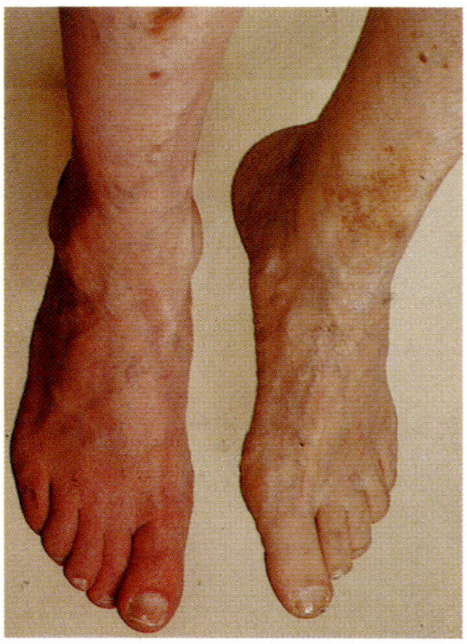

62 Rubor due to pooling of blood. The reverse of the above may be seen when the feet are hanging down—rubor on dependancy due to pooling of blood in capillaries which are dilated as a result of ischaemia. This may take a little time to develop and while it is doing so one can observe the time taken for the dorsal foot veins to fill; normal venous filling time is about 10 seconds.

63

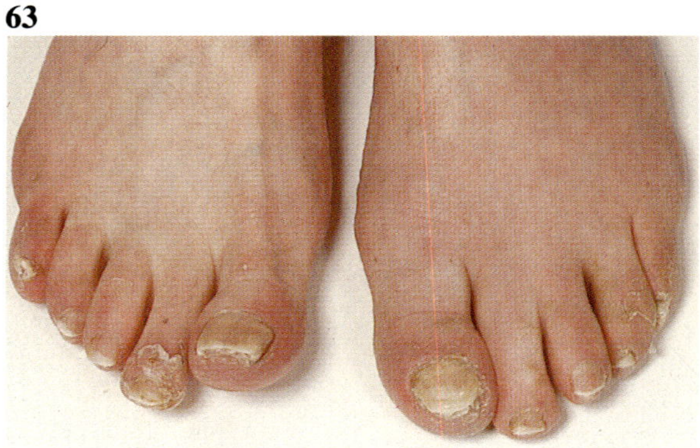

63 Limbs in ischaemic disease begin to show changes such as loss of hair (also due to tight-fitting socks), coarsening of the skin, and later thinning and ulceration as shown.

64

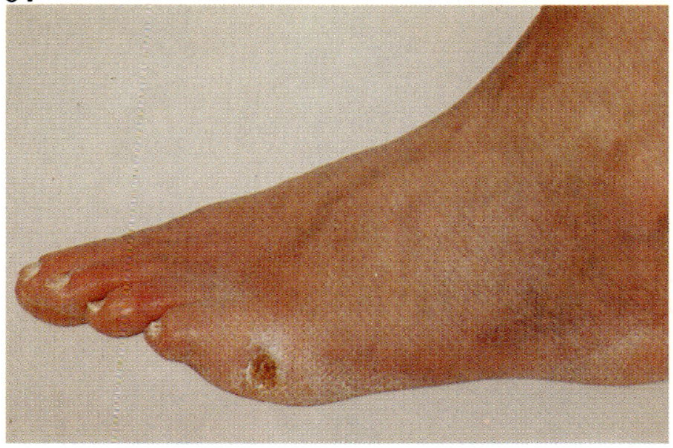

64 Pressure point ulcer. The thinning and shininess of the skin of the toes is obvious and ulceration has developed at a pressure point.

65

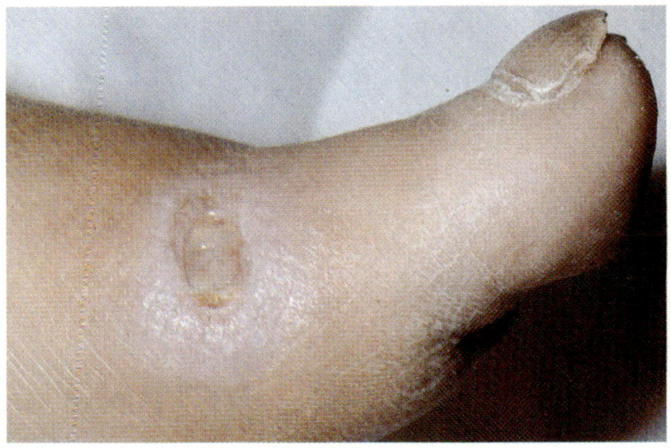

65 Pressure ischaemia. Another common site of pressure ischaemia is the 'bunion' area. The ulcers, especially in the diabetic, often penetrate deeply down to the bone.

66

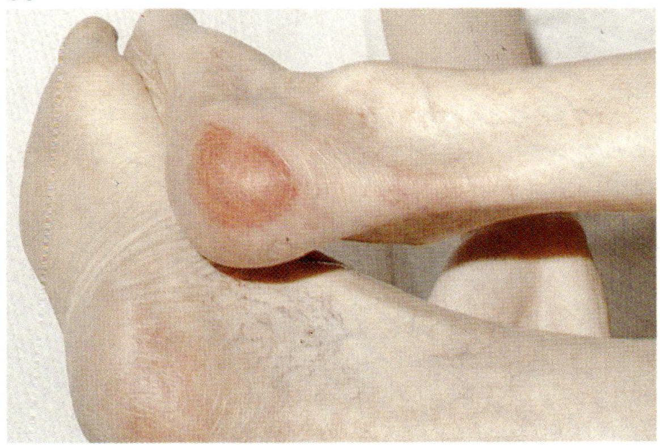

66 The heel: a pressure area. The heel is a further pressure area which may rapidly become red and painful as shown here. Later ulceration can develop and this is specially resistant to treatment. Therefore, prevention is extremely important.

67

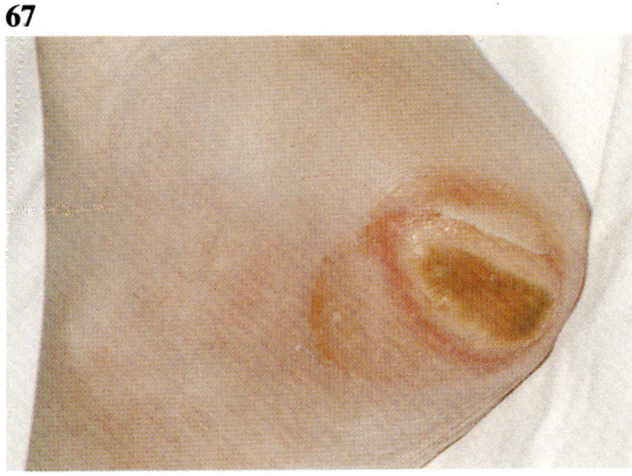

67 Ulceration of the heel has developed in this patient with severe ASO. Pain is usually a feature specially because it is difficult to avoid pressure on the area. Absence of pain usually points to diabetic ulceration.

68

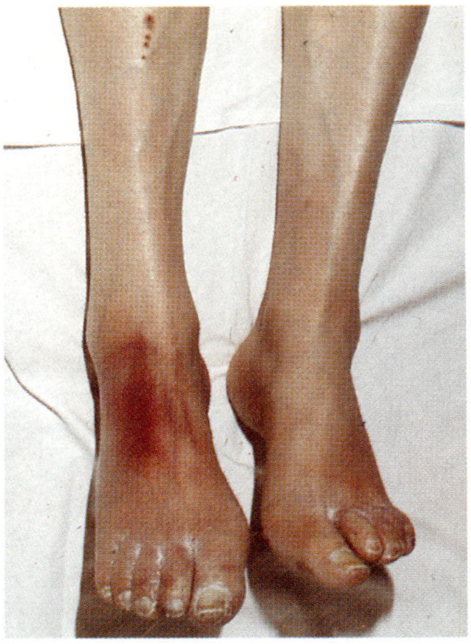

69

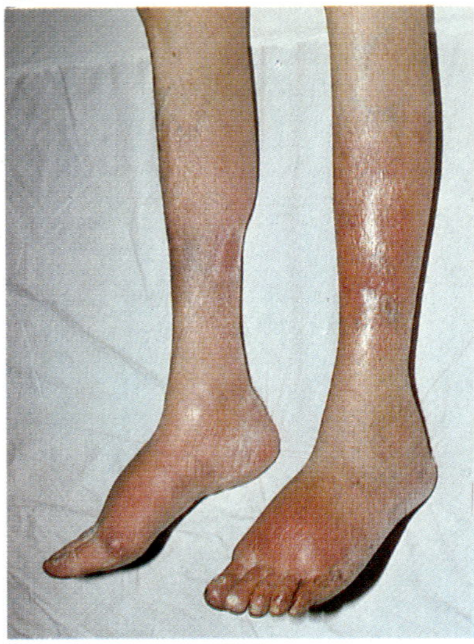

70

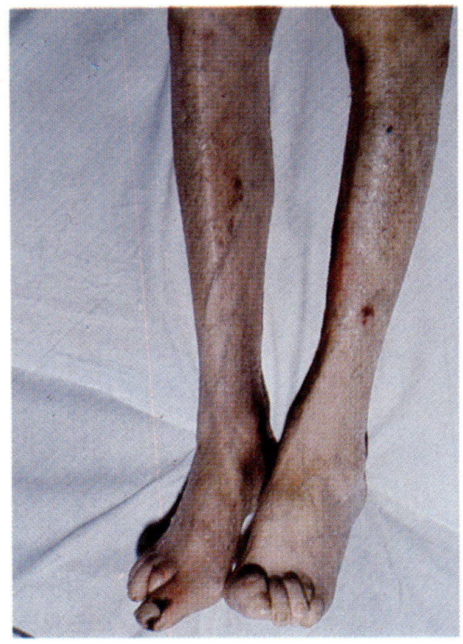

68 Reddish foot. Rest pain is often accompanied by a rather dusky reddish foot as on the right side. Hanging the foot out of bed in the cool air or placing it on the cold floor obtains pain relief.

69 Oedema of foot. With severe rest pain the frequent hanging down of the foot out of bed or sitting up all night produces oedema as in this patient's left foot, and contractures.

70 Muscle wasting in ASO. In long-standing ASO, especially of aortoiliac origin, severe muscle wasting may be present. Even in more distal arterial disease a difference in limb circumference may be measurable.

Patterns of lower limb disorders

Many special investigations are now available in the study of lower limb disorders. They are designed to demonstrate the site of occlusion of the arterial tree, the pattern of atheromatous disease in the arteries, the extent of the ischaemia, and the degree of disruption of blood flow. Pictorially we can represent most easily the value of angiography which gives an anatomical appreciation of the problem.

71

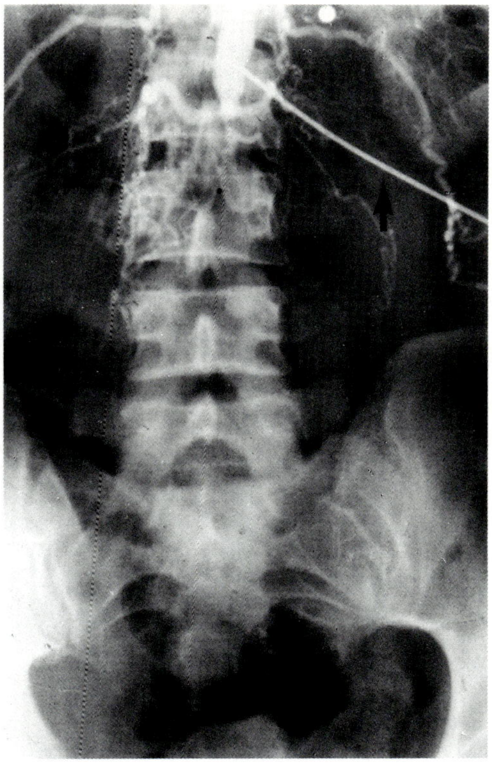

71 Percutaneous trans-lumbar aortography. Aortography can be done by a needle in the aorta as here (percutaneous trans-lumbar aortography) or by use of a Seldinger catheter passed retrogradely from the femoral artery. Narrowing of the aorta is shown at the level of the renal arteries with complete blockage below. The percutaneous needle is indicated.

72

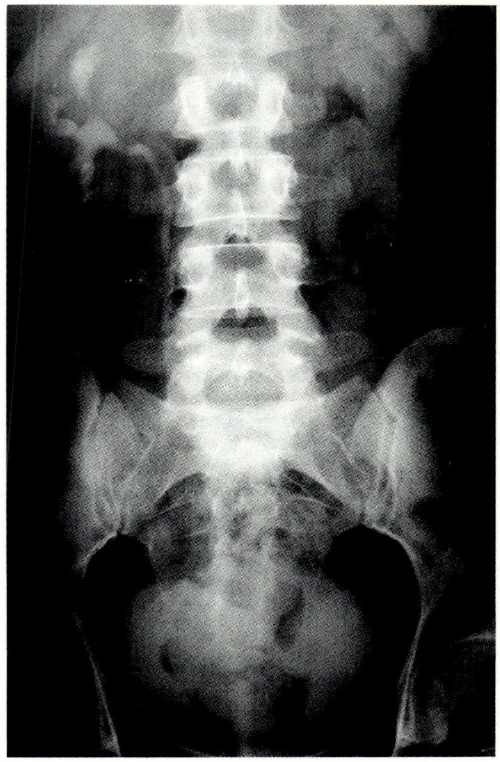

72 Intravenous pyelogram of kidney. The above patient was a 34-year-old female who presented with buttock and calf claudication at 50 metres. She had then a disobliteration of the lower aorta but the condition recurred and hypertension developed. Intravenous pyelogram showed a non-functioning of the left kidney.

73

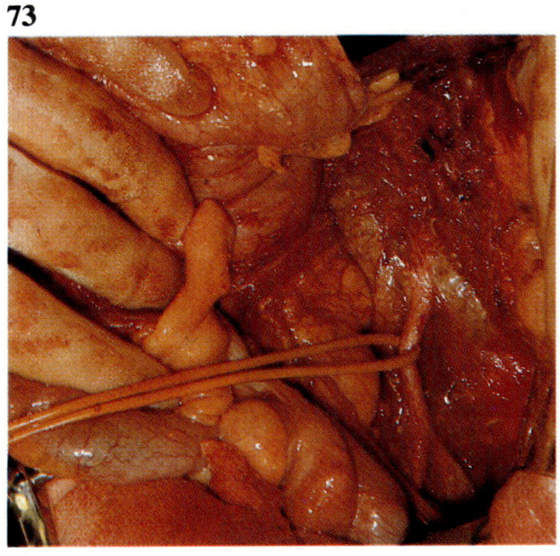

73 Narrowed iliac artery. At a second operation the aorta was hidden by fibrosis. The IVC is visible and the right common iliac artery is narrowed down to its bifurcation.

74

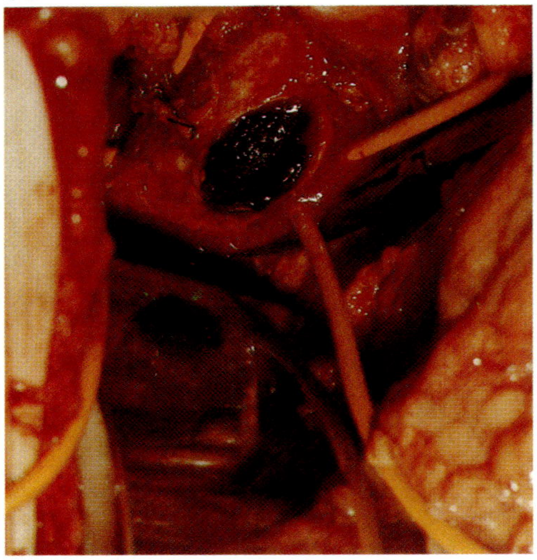

75

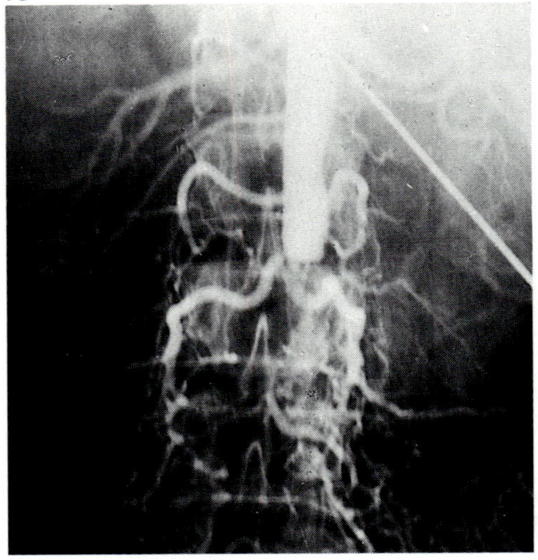

74 Aortic thrombosis. The aorta is shown opened up just below the left renal artery. A fresh thrombus is visible and below it old thrombus. An aorto-femoral bypass relieved symptoms. Aortic thrombosis in premenopausal, non-smoking women suggests a possible underlying collagen disorder. None, so far, was found in this case.

75 Obstruction of aorta. This figure shows the much more common obstruction at the lower end of the aorta in a 55-year-old man who was a heavy smoker. He had buttock and calf claudication at 50 metres and impotence—the Leriche syndrome.

76

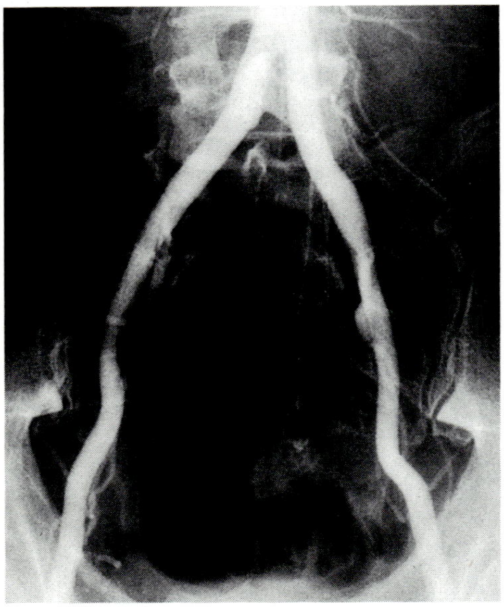

77

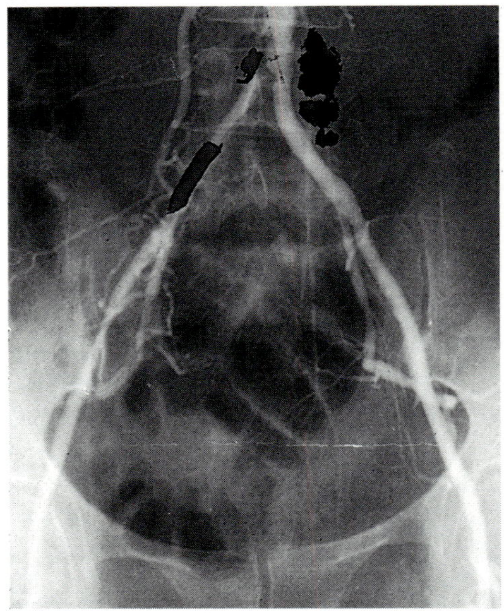

76 Stenosis and blockage of iliac arteries. Impotence due to loss of blood flow may also be seen in blockage of both internal iliac arteries. In this case in a 48-year-old man the left internal iliac artery is blocked and severe stenosis is present in the right one. Much, however, depends on the efficiency of the collateral circulation. Furthermore, the cause of impotence is difficult to assess accurately.

77 Iliac artery obstruction. A severe degree of lower aortic and right common iliac obstruction. The dark shadows are the atheromatous plaques removed by endarterectomy and laid alongside or, as in the case of the iliac artery, on the area of blockage. The right femoral pulse was absent.

78

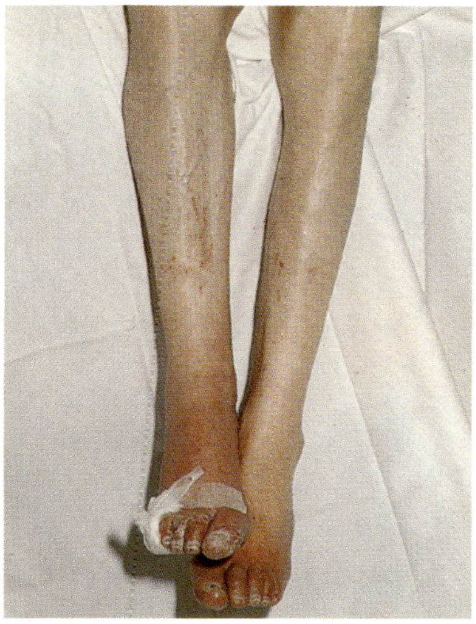

78 In aorto-iliac disease the skin is often normal in colour at rest, but with severe degrees of obstruction the legs may become cold and bluish and ulceration may develop. Gangrene is uncommon except where an occlusion of the femoral artery is also present.

79

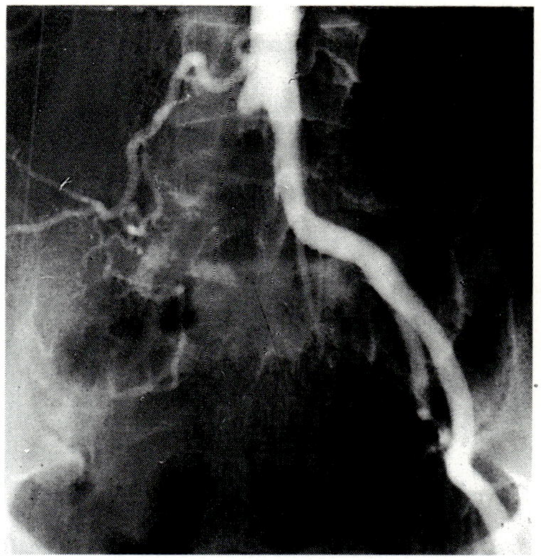

79 Occluded iliac arteries. The iliac arteries in the right leg were completely occluded, extending right down to the popliteal artery which was very narrowed. The patient had a very severely ischaemic limb with gangrene of the foot.

80

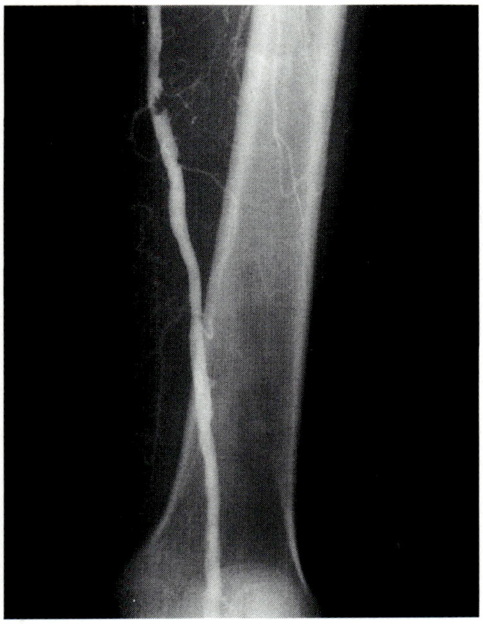

80 Narrowing of femoral artery. The commonest form of intermittent claudication occurs in the calf and is caused by obstruction of the femoral artery. This usually begins in the region of the adductor magnus opening. A short segment narrowing is shown.

81

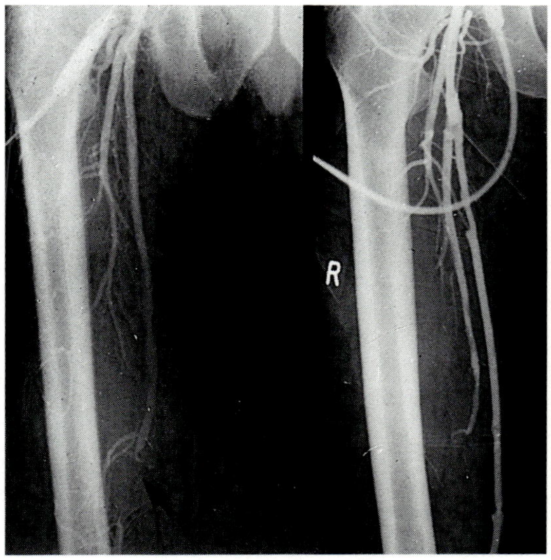

81 Obstruction of femoral artery. The obstruction elongates by progressive thrombosis and organisation up to the beginning of the superficial femoral artery. The plate on the left shows a long obstruction of the superficial femoral artery. The profunda femoris crosses the femur at the junction of the upper and middle third. On the right is the postoperative result with a reversed saphenous graft in position.

82

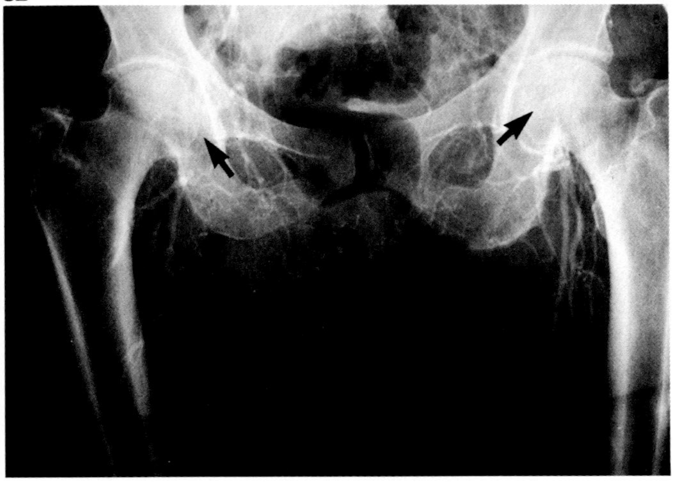

82 Occlusion of the common femoral artery–in this case both—is less common and occurs in about 10 per cent of cases. As it narrows it obliterates the profunda femoris as well as the superficial femoral artery, so that the clinical features are severe with gangrene a common feature.

83

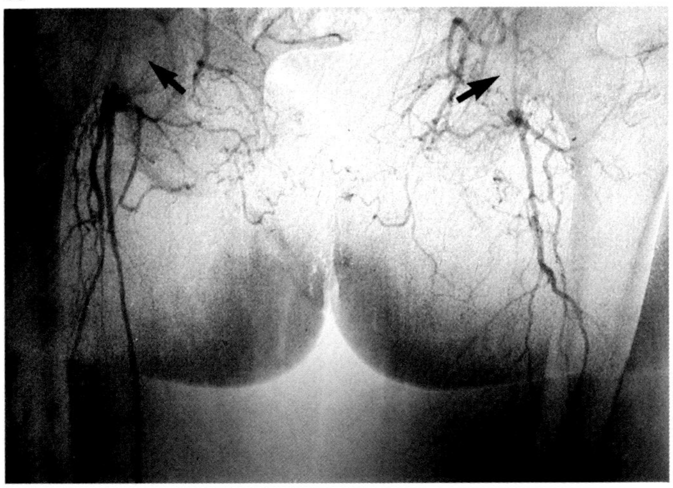

83 Occlusion of femoral artery. This is a negative of the above which tends to show more clearly the degree of obstruction being greater on the left side.

84

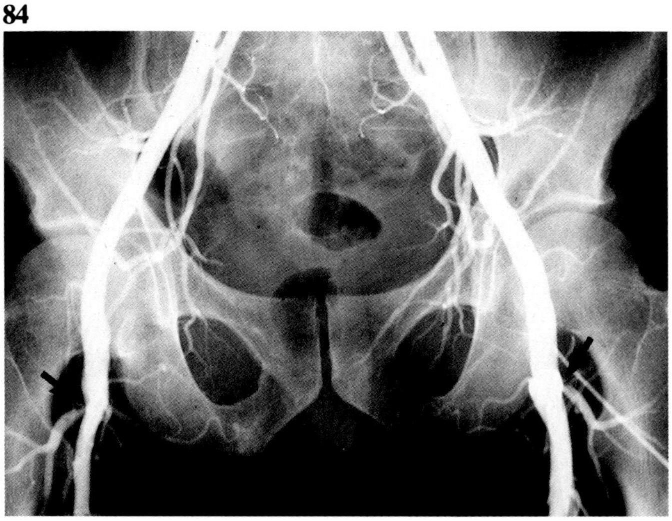

84 Stenosis of the origins of both profunda femoris arteries are seen in this film. It is important to determine this as in the event of the superficial femoral being blocked, limb survival really depends on the profunda flow.

85

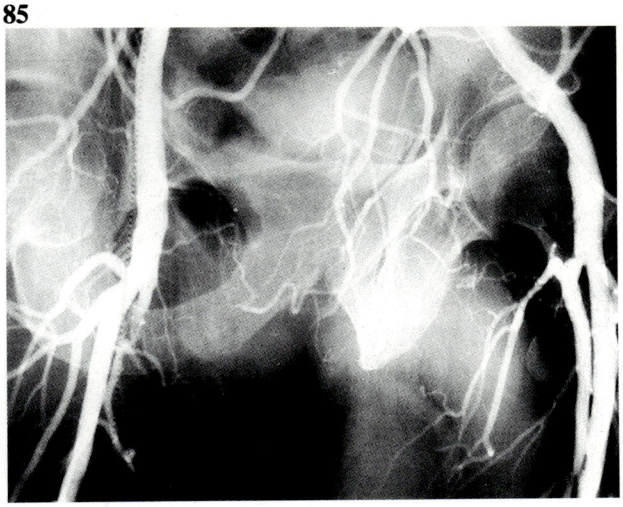

85 Collar-type stenosis. A lateral or oblique view is often necessary to get a good view of the origin of the profunda artery which lies posterior to the common femoral. Otherwise a collar-type stenosis of the origin may be missed.

86

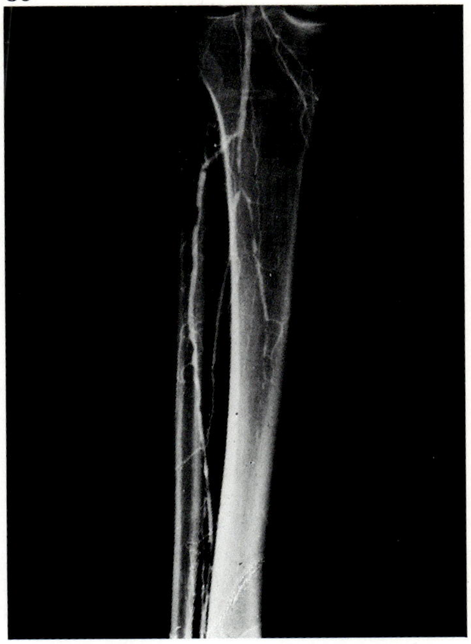

86 Segmental blockage of vessels. The run off or patency of the three vessels below the knee (anterior tibial, posterior tibial, and peroneal) is important to assess with regard to value of grafts and prognosis as regards limb survival. At least one main vessel should be patent. This shows segmental blocking of the three vessels.

87

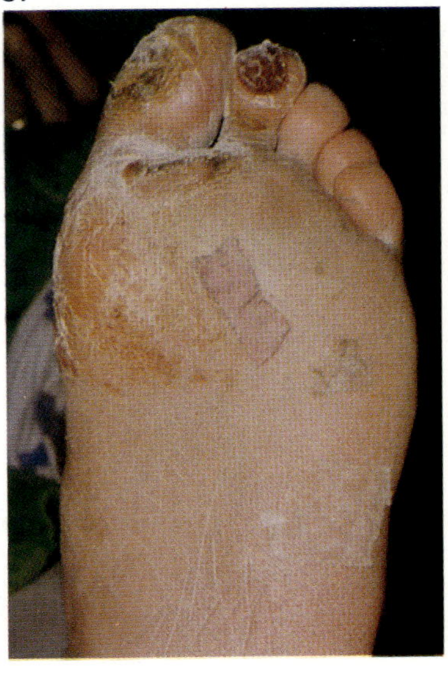

87 Distal ASO disease. This 54-year-old patient has the typical ulceration and gangrene of the toes specially seen in the diabetic with more pronounced distal ASO disease.

88

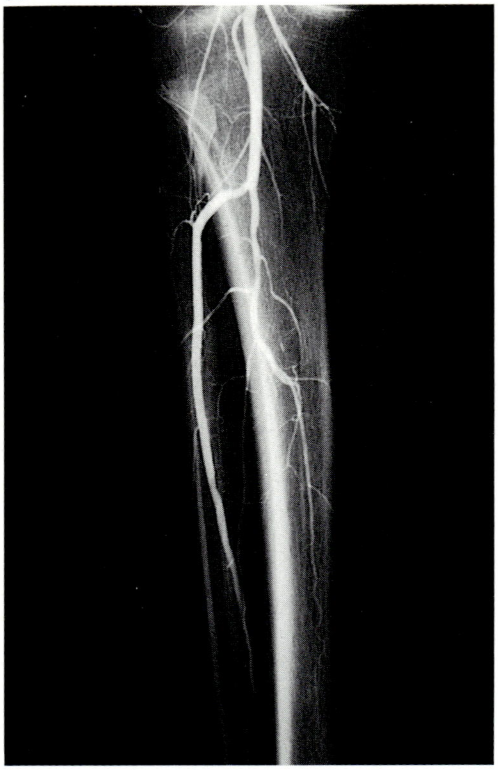

88 **Normal popliteal artery.** In the above the vessels down to the popliteal bifurcation were normal. The anterior tibial artery on the left of the picture tapers off as it passes down the limb. The other two vessels stop about mid-calf.

89

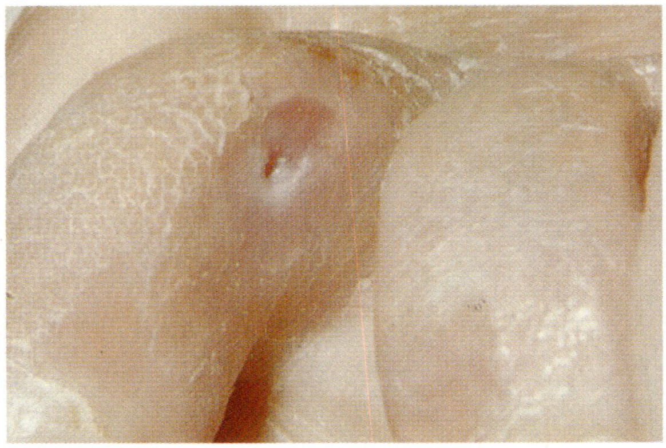

89 **Diabetic necrosis.** Ulceration between the toes is another common area of necrosis in the diabetic. These may not be painful if a diabetic neuropathy is present. The ulceration may extend down to the bone or into a joint.

90

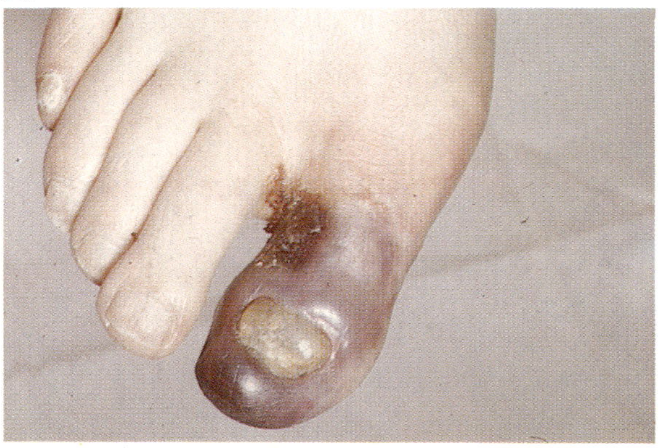

90 **Gangrene in the big toe** may come on gradually in ASO. Sometimes as a result of trauma, even that of simple chiropody where infection may supervene. The rest of the foot is pale. Arteriogram showed complete block in the femoral artery and the anterior tibial artery.

91

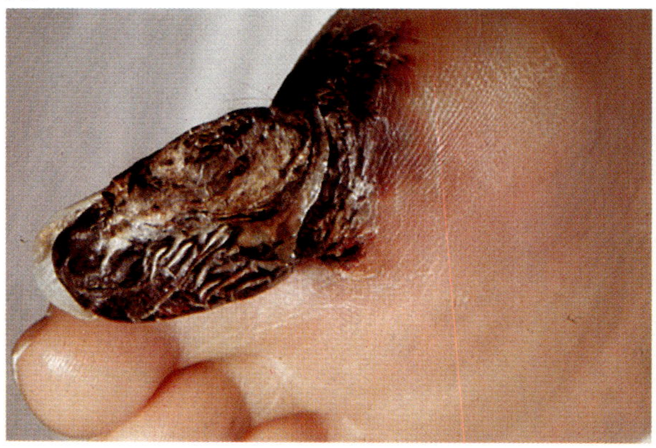

91 **Mummification of toe.** The gangrene may progress to mummification of the toe which can slough off. Extension of the gangrene beyond the base into the forefoot will possibly require a forefoot amputation but more likely a below-knee type in a non-diabetic.

92

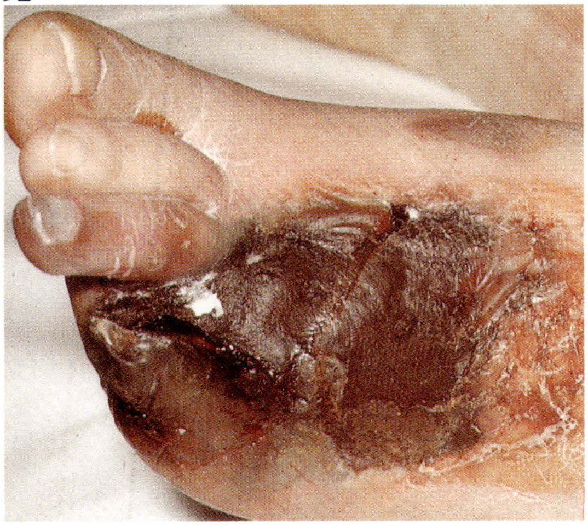

92 Moist gangrene. When infection occurs in relation to gangrene the moist form is seen especially in the diabetic. In this 54-year-old man, a diabetic and heavy smoker, the vessels below the knee were obliterated and a below-knee amputation was necessary.

93

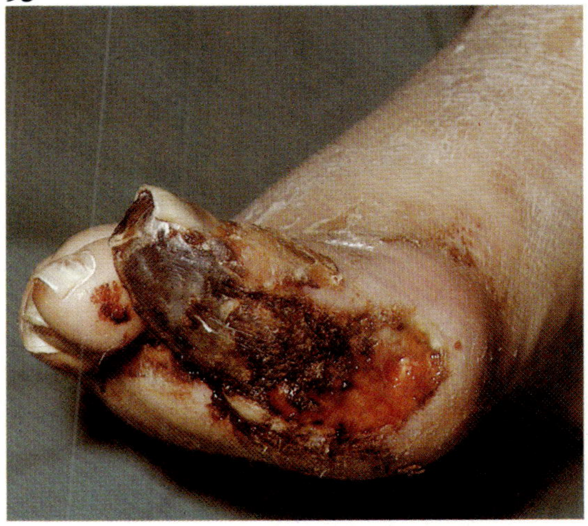

93 Diabetic gangrene. In the diabetic and indeed every elderly person care must be taken with the feet. Over-enthusiastic chiropody, especially by the untrained, may allow infection into an area of balanced ischaemia and lead to gangrene. This patient dug into the side of the nail with scissors. A part foot amputation was successful.

94

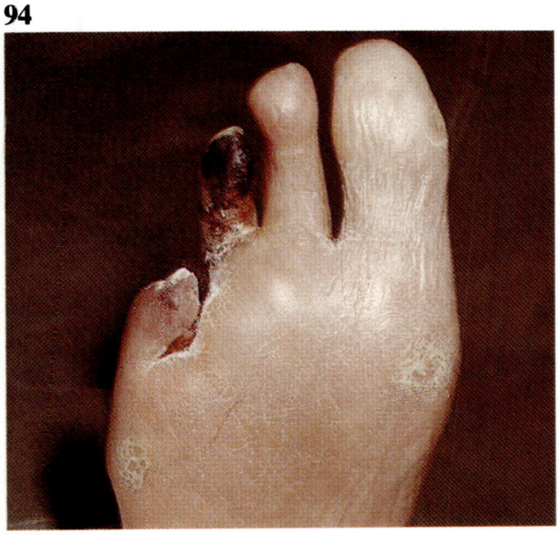

94 Lateral toe gangrene. Although the big toe is often affected by gangrene, other toes especially the lateral ones may suffer.

95

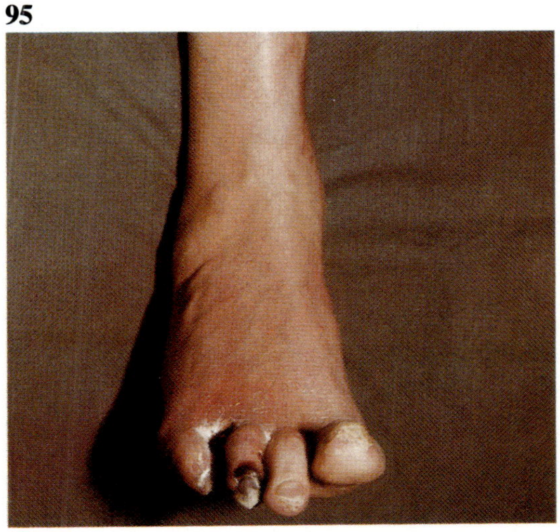

95 Rubor of stasis. When the above foot was photographed in the dependent position the rubor of stasis was clearly evident. In this case a below knee amputation was required.

96

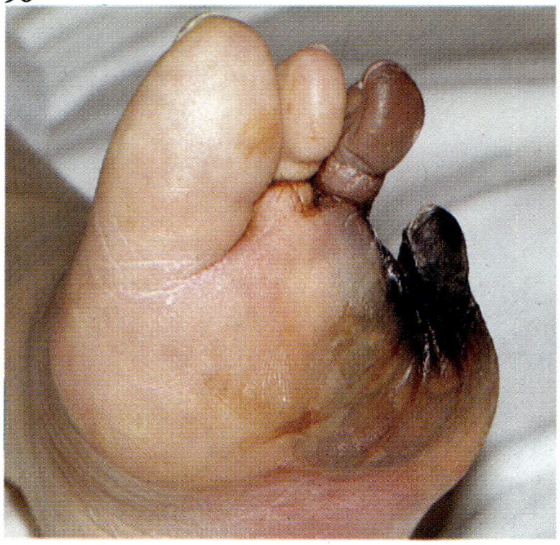

97

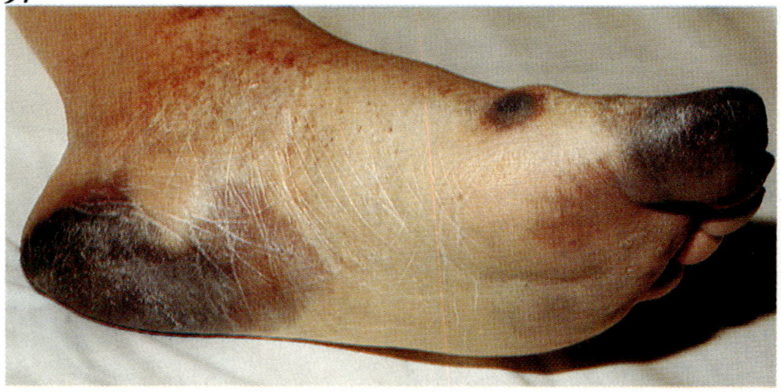

97 Ischaemic heel. Apart from the toes, another important area that suffers in the ischaemic foot is the heel and outer border of the foot where they are allowed to press on the bed for hours.

96 Dry gangrene. This diabetic patient had a local amputation of the fourth toe for dry gangrene. Infection and a nasty moist gangrene followed. If operative trauma can be followed by infection, how much more careful must we be with non-professional foot care.

98

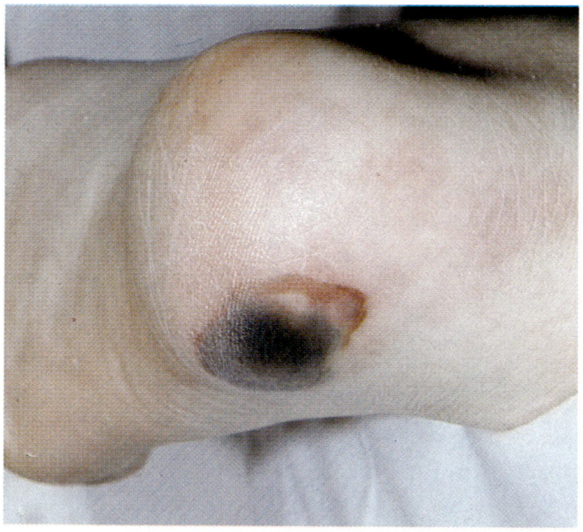

99

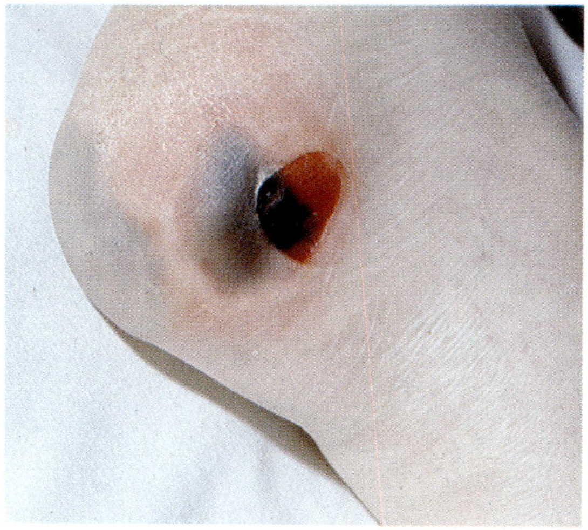

98 Superficial pressure gangrene of heel. A less severe form of this superficial gangrene due to pressure. The skin separates in time and an ulcer is left which is often painful. Even pressure on the heel for a short time, while lying on the operating table, may lead to this condition and cause much suffering.

99 Pressure-damaged heel. This figure shows the appearance a few days later in the above female patient. When one compares this with the previous picture there is no indication that the heel was damaged and yet it must have been. One cannot overemphasise the care of the heels as well as the toes in the elderly, and even in the middle aged, where the peripheral circulation may be impaired.

4 Cerebrovascular disease

100

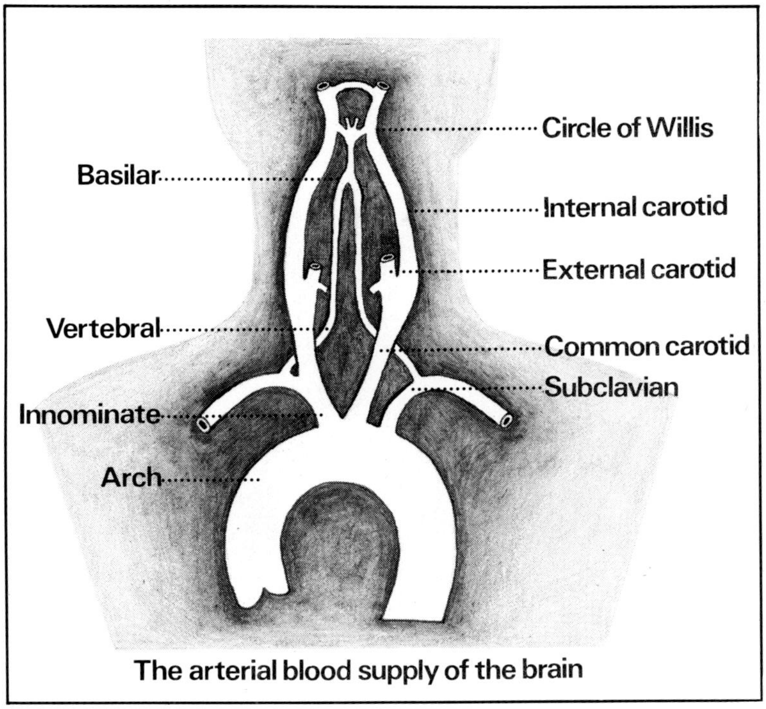

100 Arterial blood supply to brain. This schematic diagram demonstrates the arterial blood supply to the brain. The outlined figure is not exact with reference to division of the vessels. Occlusions, single or multiple, from the aortic arch upwards may influence the blood supply to the brain.

101

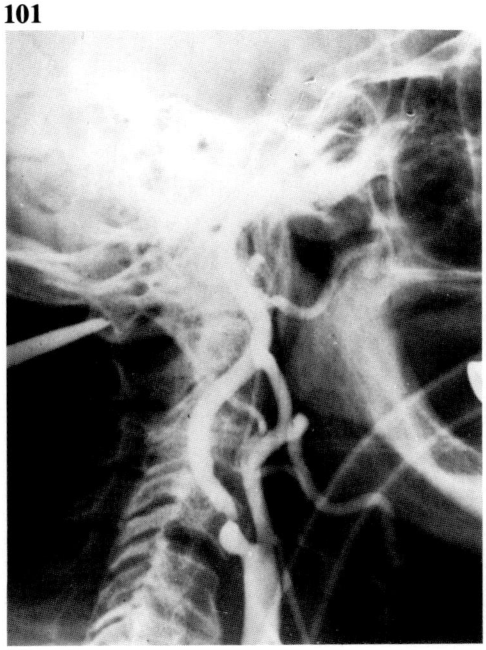

101 Stenosis of the internal carotid artery is shown and is due to ASO. The clinical features are transient ischaemic attacks (TIA), with muscle weakness of the contralateral limbs. A thrill may be palpated over the artery and a bruit heard. Arch aortography will exclude a lesion of the arch and proximal vessels, and angiography of the carotid will demonstrate the lesion.

102

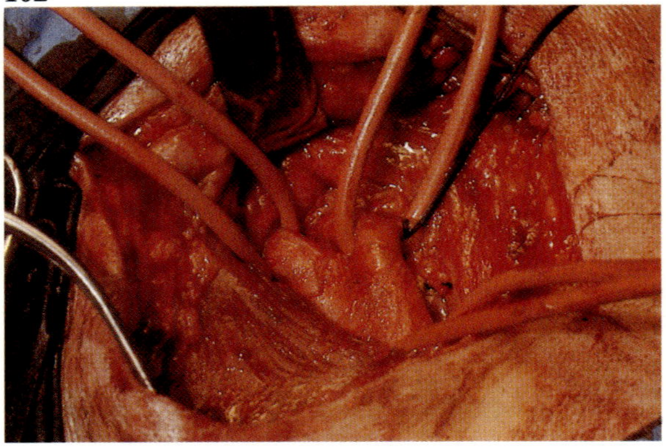

102 Atheroma of internal carotid artery. The common carotid artery and its division is visible. The medial branch is the external carotid artery marked by a silk tie on its first branch. Lateral is the internal carotid artery with the atheroma in its wall giving a yellowish-red appearance.

103

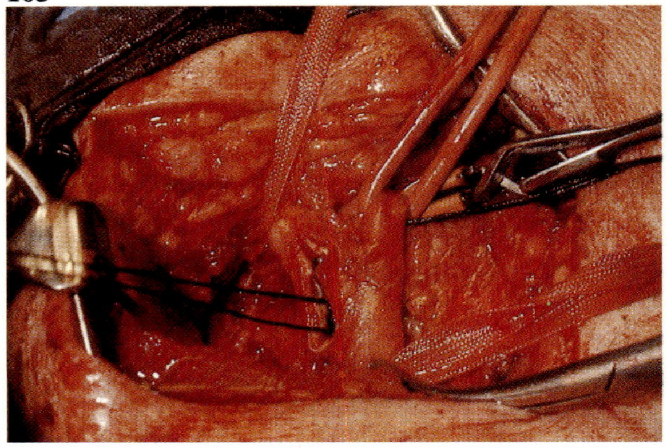

103 Removal of atheroma. The internal carotid artery is opened up. Inside is an internal shunt placed to allow continuous blood flow while the atheroma is being removed. This may be as a smooth plaque or it may be ulcerated and local thrombosis may be present. Symptoms may be due to microemboli arising from the plaque.

104

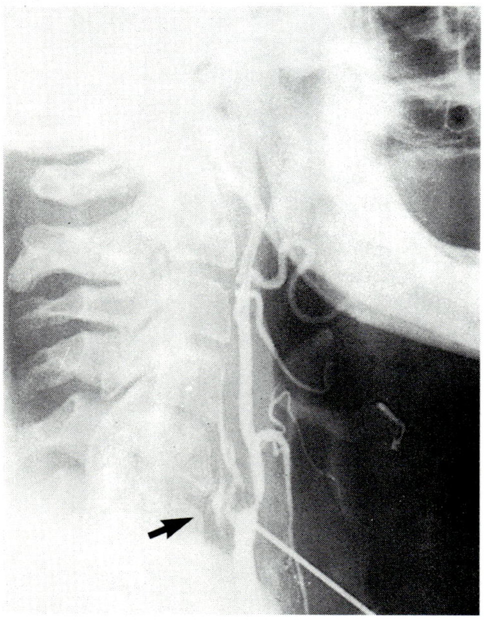

104 Occlusion of internal carotid artery. On occasion a complete occlusion of the internal carotid artery may have occurred. This is inoperable.

105

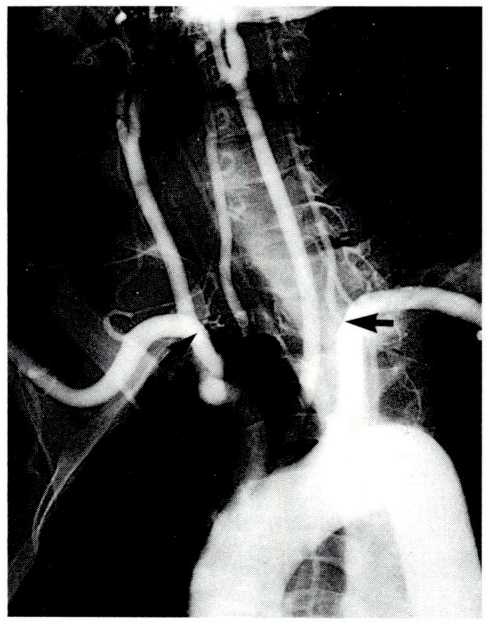

105 Vertebral artery stenosis may cause 'drop attacks' due to ischaemia of the hind brain. In such cases the patient may feel sick, and develop weakness of one side of the body which may cause him to fall to that side. Recovery takes place in a few minutes. A bruit may be heard in the base of the neck. Diagnosis is confirmed by arch aortography. Note absence of right vertebral artery and narrowing of the origin of the left one.

106

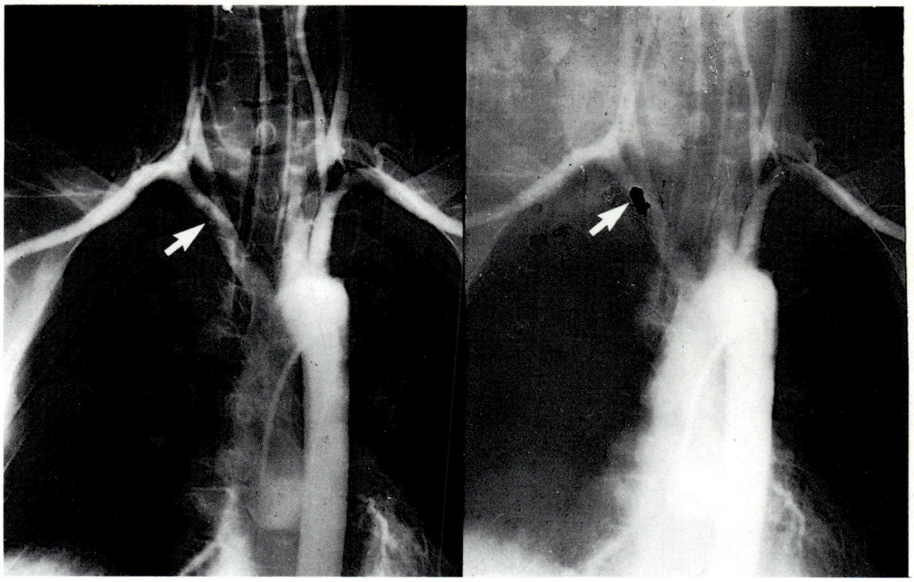

106 Stenosis of the subclavian artery usually occurs near its origin and may produce claudication in the arm muscles. The blood pressure on the affected side is less than the other. An atheromatous plaque is present in the right subclavian artery in the left picture. On the right picture the removed plaque is superimposed on the arteriogram.

107

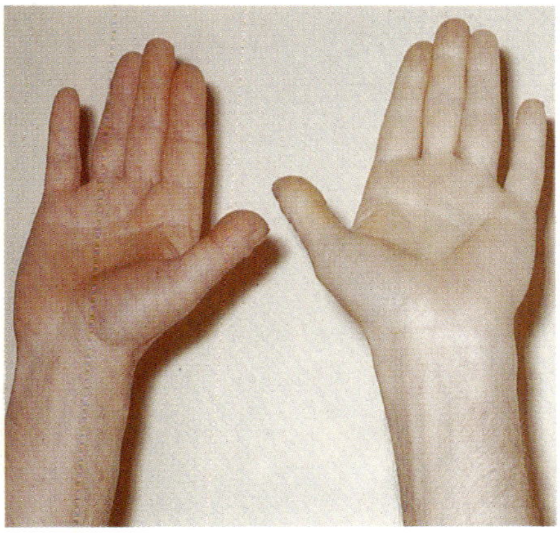

107 Claudication of the forearm muscles may be accompanied, as in the lower limb, by coldness and pallor of the hand. This is well shown here and is sometimes taken as Raynaud's syndrome but of the unilateral variety.

108

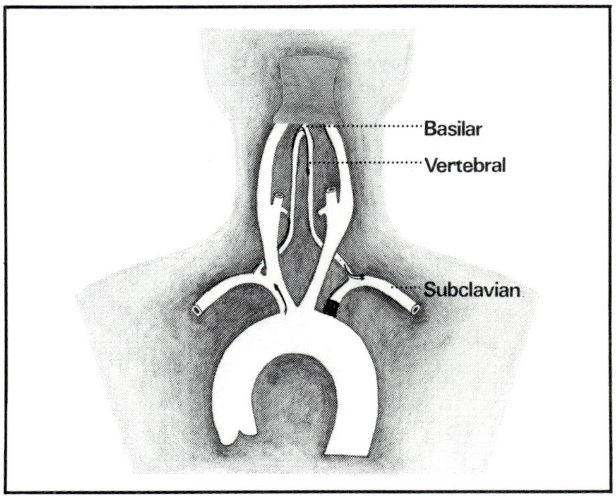

108 Vertebrobasilar insufficiency. A complete block of the subclavian artery may give rise to the subclavian steal syndrome which is really vertebrobasilar insufficiency due to a demand for blood to the upper limb being met with reversed flow down the vertebral artery.

109

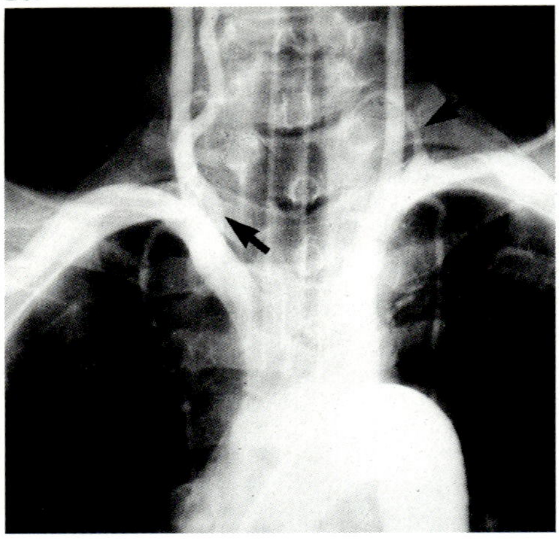

110

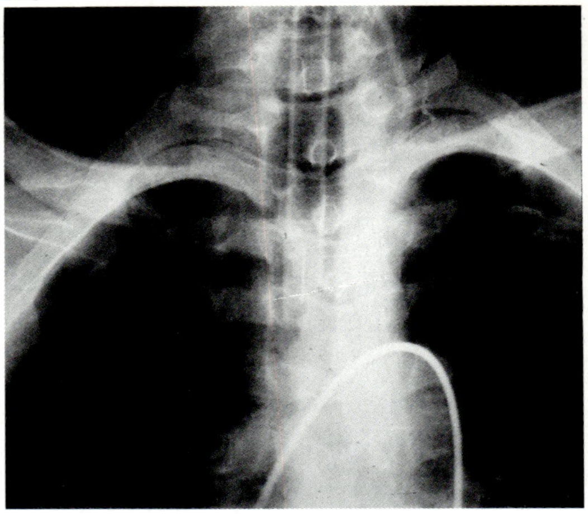

109 Narrowing of the left subclavian artery is not easy to visualise in this film because of the imposition of the common carotid artery. The right vertebral is clearly visible and well filled; the left vertebral is poorly visualised.

110 Retrograde flow in vertebral artery. This is a late film demonstrating the steal. The right vertebral artery is not visible but flow is still present in the left vertebral artery, i.e. retrograde flow. A graft was placed between the common carotid and the left subclavian artery eliminating the need for retrograde flow.

Thoracic aorta

111

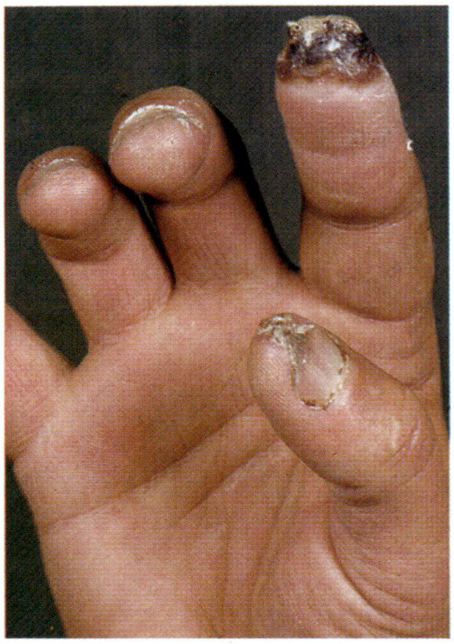

112

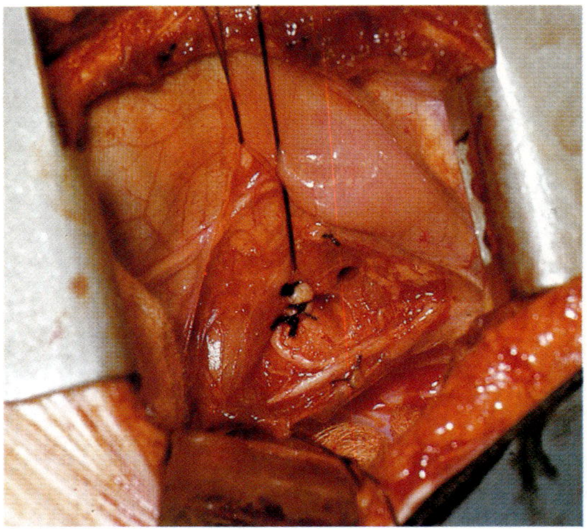

112 Patent ductus arteriosus. This vessel passes between the pulmonary artery and the arch or descending aorta. It is picked up in infants and children with heart failure and a machinery type murmur is heard over the pulmonary area. The ductus is shown with silk ties round it. The vagus nerve is visible with the recurrent laryngeal nerve curving round the lower margin of the ductus.

111 Partial occlusion of the subclavian artery was found on aortography in this patient who developed embolic gangrene of the index finger and thumb. He had unilateral Raynaud's syndrome on this side previously. The emboli originated from an ulcerated atheromatous plaque.

113

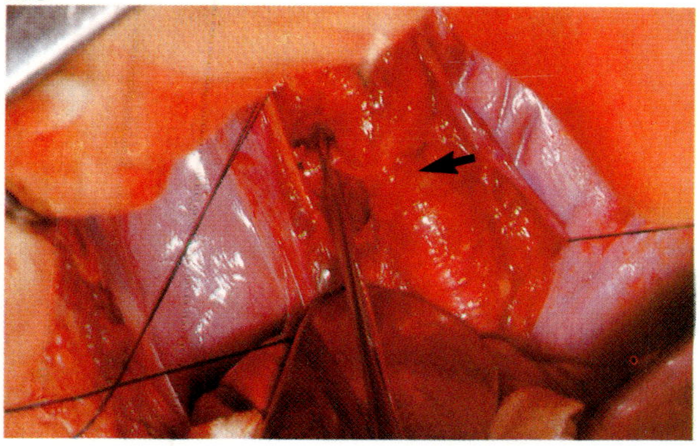

113 Coarctation of the aorta is a congenital narrowing at or below the origin of the ductus. Hypertension may occur above the narrowing and hypotension below. The femoral pulses are absent. The ductus is clamped and below it the aorta shows a narrow waist.

114

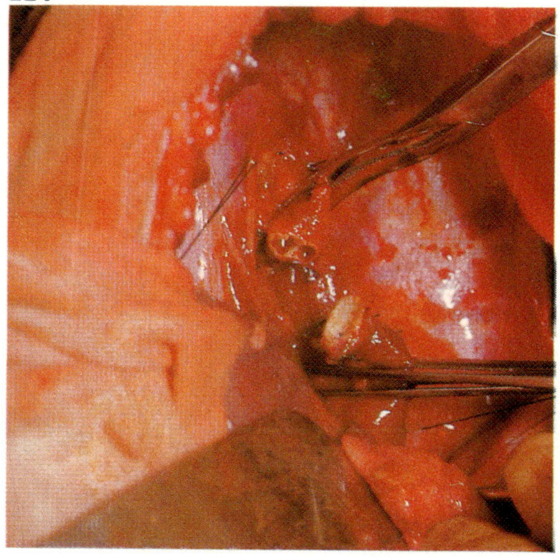

114 Divided aorta. The aorta has been divided at the level of the ductus. The artery held in the upper clamp shows the double lumen (ductus and aorta). A tiny pinhole opening is just visible at level of coarctation.

115

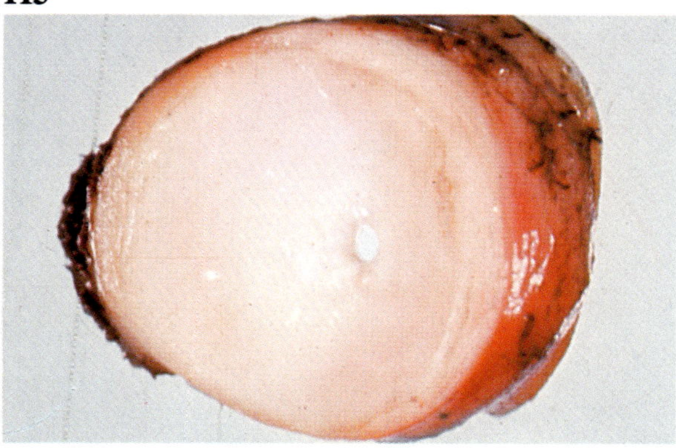

115 Aorta: resected specimen. The resected specimen with the very small eccentrically sited opening. At operation tortuous dilated collateral vessels were seen above the coarctation and can cause notching of the ribs on plain x-ray.

116

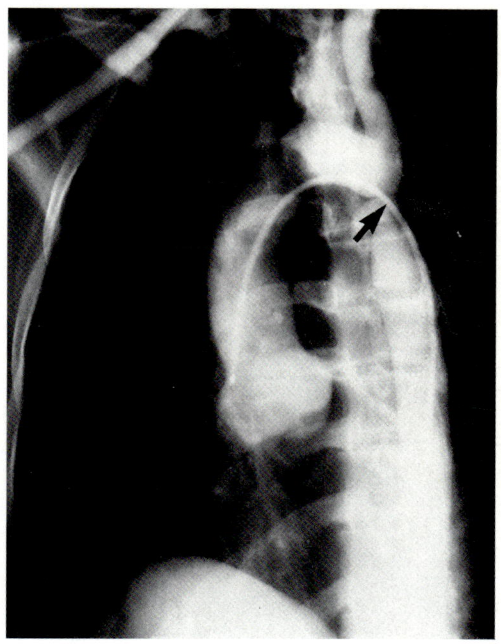

116 Narrowing of aorta. Aortography demonstrates the narrowing of the aorta below the level of the left subclavian artery.

117

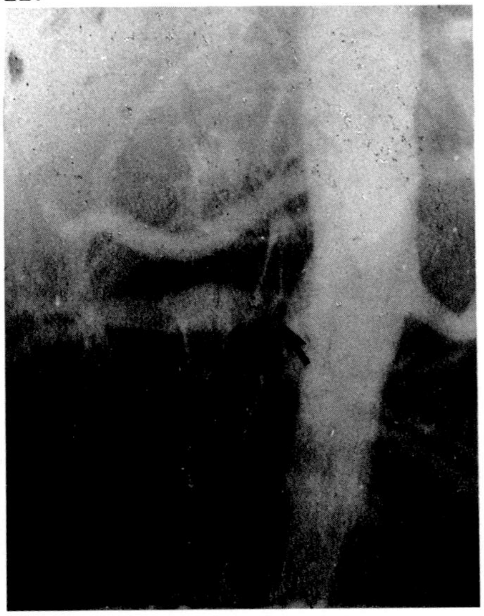

118

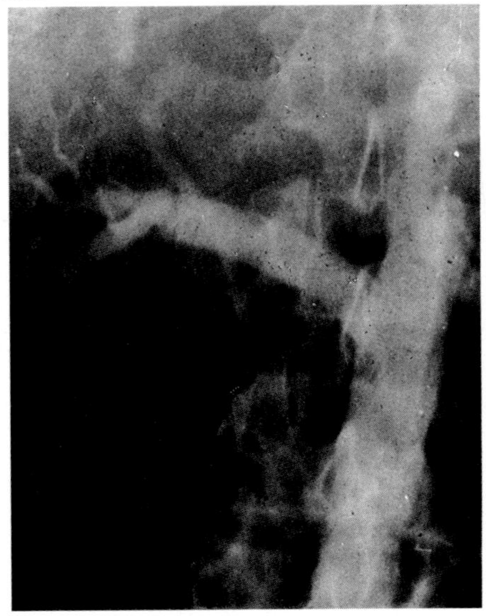

117 Renal artery stenosis is nearly always due to ASO or fibromuscular hyperplasia. Other causes are rare. Clinically the patient may present with hypertension and a bruit may be heard close to the umbilicus on the affected side. Although a number of investigative procedures are available, aortography demonstrates the anatomy of the problem. The right renal artery is narrowed at its origin due to ASO in a 52-year-old man. Post-stenotic dilatation is demonstrated.

118 Surgical treatment of renal artery stenosis. A variety of procedures is used in the surgical treatment from nephrectomy, endarterectomy, splenorenal anastomosis to bypass grafts. This patient had a Dacron graft inserted between the renal artery and the aorta, as shown in this arteriogram.

119

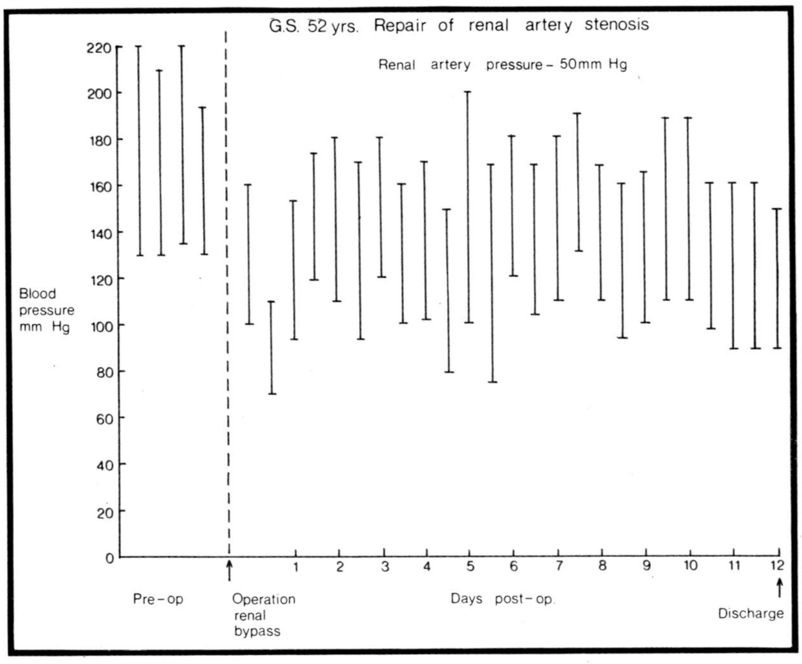

119 Surgery in hypertension. Although the results of surgery in reduction of hypertension is rather disappointing, this patient did well. When seen a year later the pressure was still down. Antihypertensive drugs have now replaced surgery.

Ischaemic syndromes in the gut

The intestines are supplied by three main arteries, coeliac axis, superior and inferior mesenteric with also support from the internal iliac arteries. Such is the profusion of interconnections that it usually requires two of the three main arteries to be occluded to produce symptoms. Sudden occlusion of the superior mesenteric vessels, however, can produce acute symptoms.

120

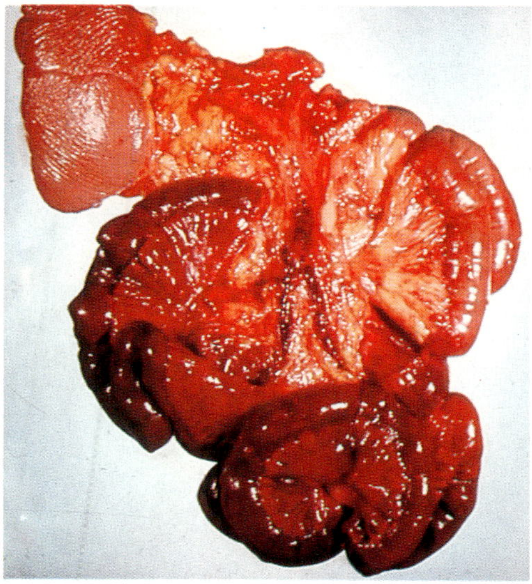

120 An arterial embolus or thrombosis of the superior mesenteric artery or vein can produce widespread ischaemia and gangrene of the gut. Clinical features are sudden onset of abdominal pain, minimal tenderness and a high leucocytosis. A bloody diarrhoea may also be present. Diagnosis is established by operation.

121

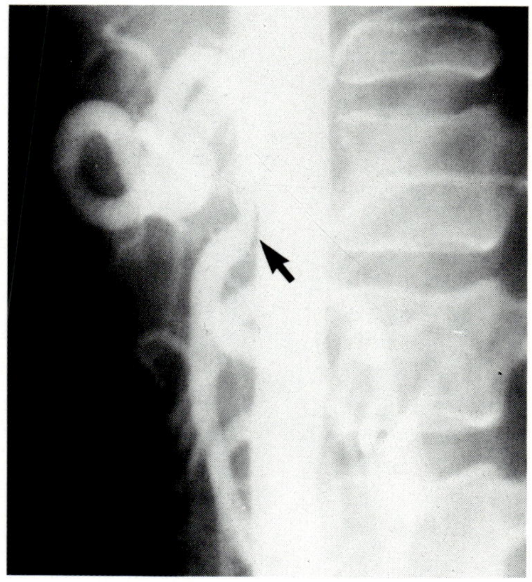

121 Chronic occlusion of the arteries may be due to atheroma at the aortic origin or possibly external compression. Clinical features are colicky abdominal pain within 30 minutes after a meal. Because eating causes pain weight loss is a feature. A bruit may be heard in the epigastric region. Arteriography may show, as here, narrowing of the origin of the superior mesenteric artery due to atheroma.

122

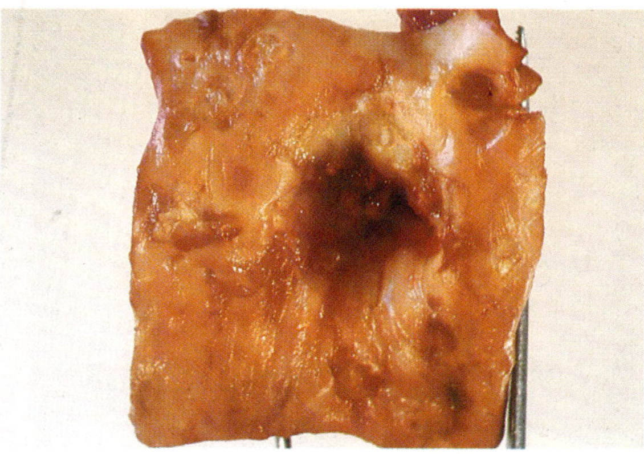

122 Mesenteric artery narrowing. Narrowing of the opening of the superior mesenteric artery is visualised from an open aorta. Thrombus is present in the lumen.

123

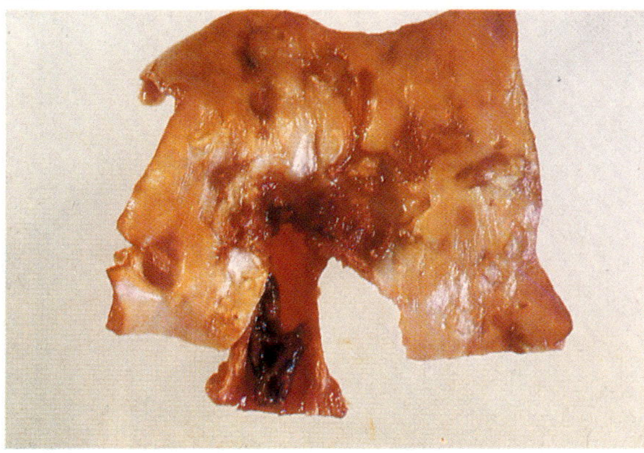

123 The superior mesenteric artery is opened into the aorta. Thrombus is present and the atheromatous collar round the origin is clearly visible.

124

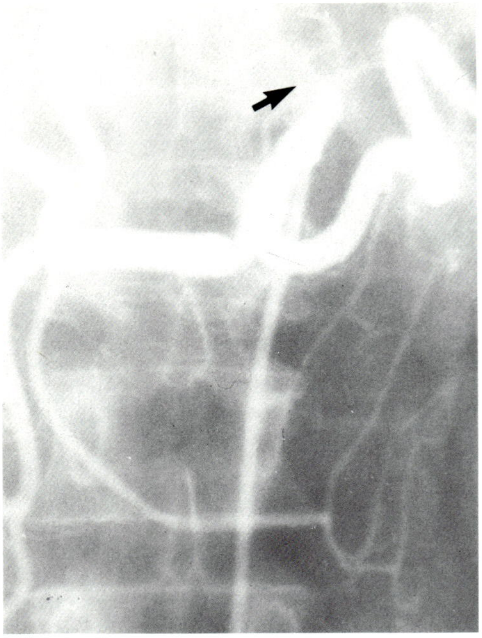

124 Coeliac axis compression is perhaps a doubtful entity where abdominal angina is related to compression of the coeliac axis origin by a band. The aortogram suggests narrowing of the origin of the axis—possibly atheroma due to atheroma or external pressure.

125

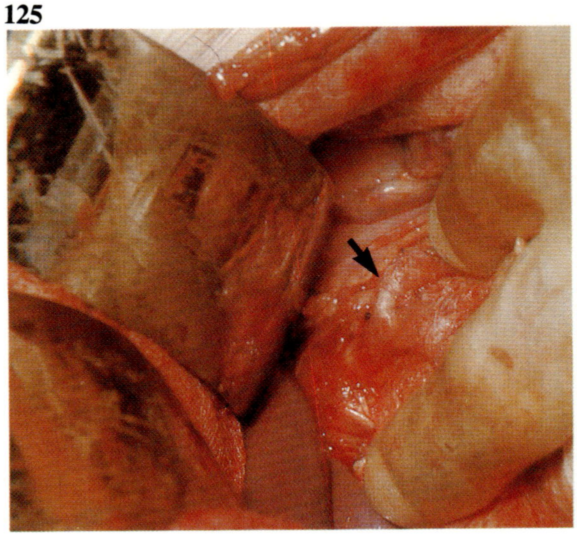

125 Compression of coeliac axix. At operation the median arcuate ligament seemed to be compressing the coeliac axis. The pressure and wave forms in the branch of the artery were same as in the aorta. Median ligament was divided but abdominal pain was unchanged.

126

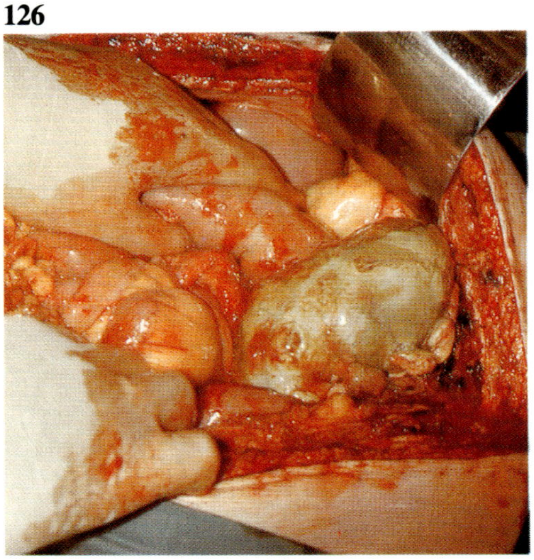

126 Sigmoid colon gangrene. Division of the inferior mesenteric artery is necessary in resection of an abdominal aortic aneurysm. In a few instances gangrene of the sigmoid colon may result as shown here due to poor collateral circulation.

127

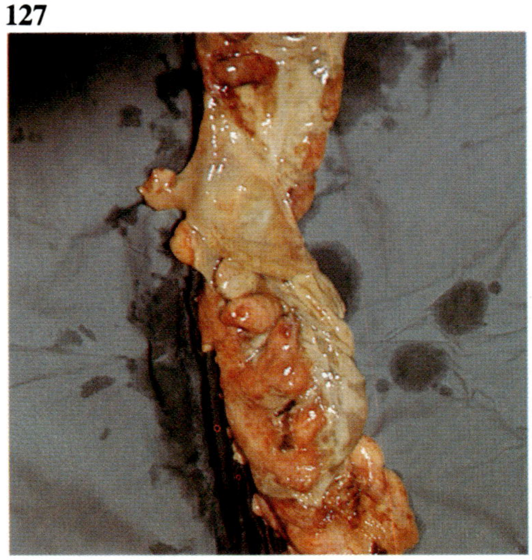

127 Resected bowel in colon gangrene. A portion of the resected bowel removed in above case. The colon had to be removed from splenic flexure to anus. The patient developed diarrhoea on the third postoperative day. Proctoscopy may help in diagnosis but laparotomy should not be delayed. Better a needless laparotomy than miss a gangrenous bowel.

5 Aneurysms

Aneurysms are by custom defined as dilatation of a portion of the arterial wall due to disease or injury.

Classification

True	**False**
Dilatation of all coats of artery due to disease	No arterial tissue in wall Trauma
Congenital—Marfan's syndrome Ehlers-Danlos syndrome Berry aneurysm	Injury—gunshot wound knife glass
Acquired Arteriosclerosis Syphilis Post-stenotic Mycotic Arteritides	Surgery—arteriotomy grafts disc operation

128

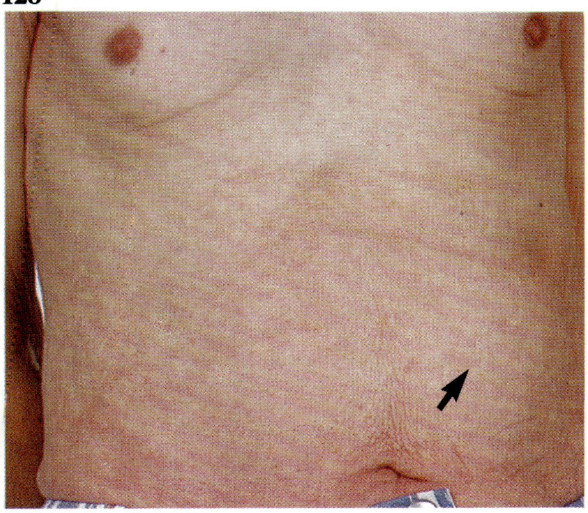

128 Aneurysm of abdominal aorta is nearly always due to arteriosclerosis obliterans (ASO). It may be asymptomatic or appear as a painless throbbing abdominal mass. It is felt above the umbilicus and has characteristic expansile pulsation. It normally bulges to the left. This feature is suggested perhaps by the slight prominence above and lateral to the umbilicus.

129

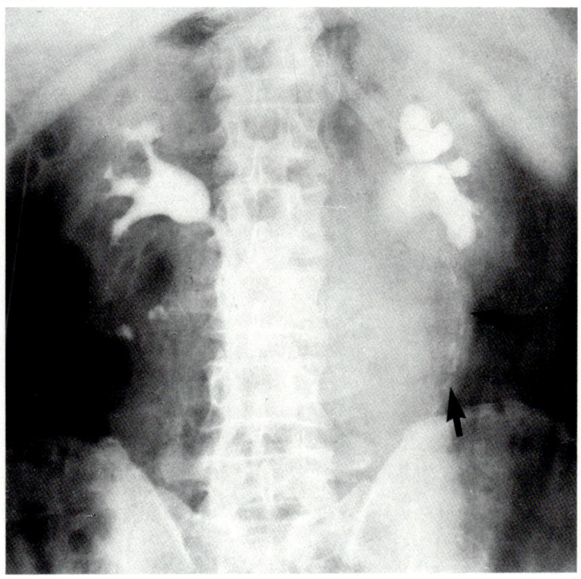

129 Calcification in wall of aorta. Confirmation of the clinical suspicion may come from x-ray of the abdomen which will show a line of calcification in the wall of the aorta, specially in the lateral view. The IVP also shows dilatation of left renal pelvis.

130

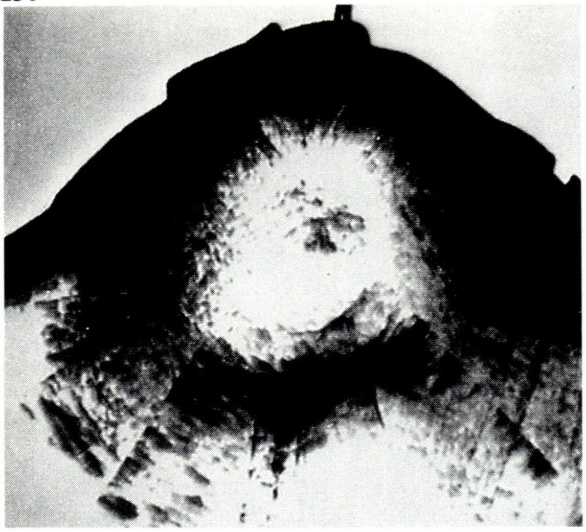

130 Aneurysm of aorta. Ultrasound is becoming an important non-invasive technique of demonstrating a central mass, its size and its progress with time. The white area in the picture represents the aneurysm, the dark area within the lumen of the aorta.

131

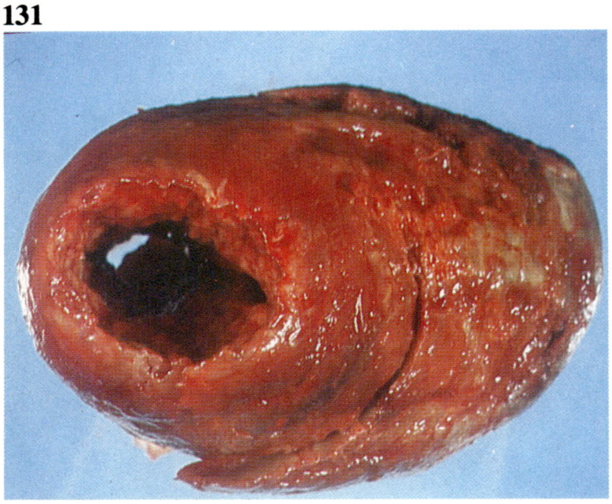

131 The bulk of the aneurysm is laminated blood clot with a small passage-way corresponding nearly to the original size of the aorta.

132

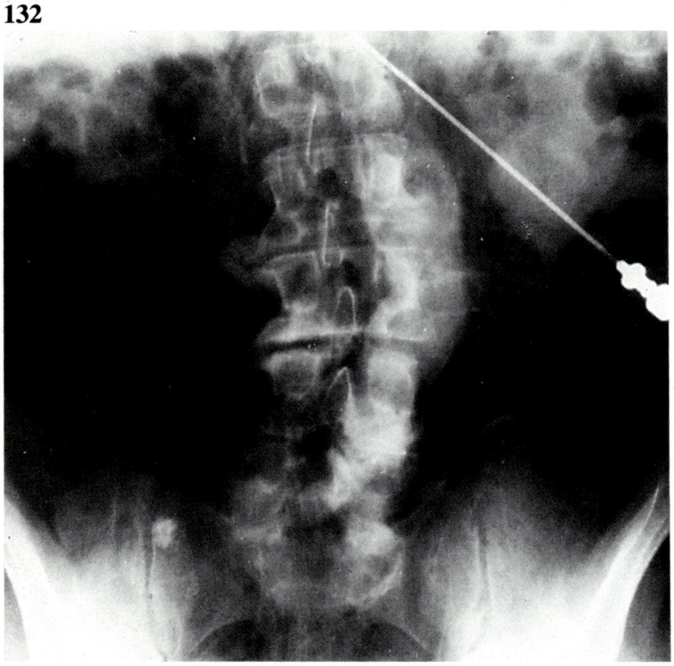

132 Abdominal aneurysms. Over 90 per cent of abdominal aneurysms originate below the renal arteries. If it is suspected that an aneurysm may involve these arteries an aortogram may be done. This will show the irregular channel in the midst of the clot.

133

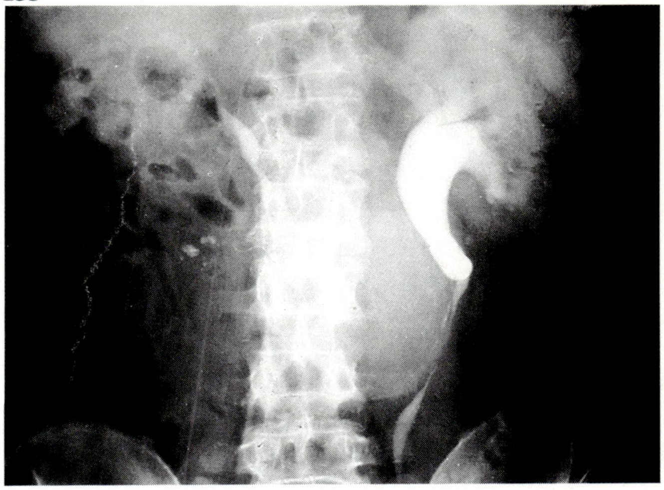

133 In the very large aneurysms the ureter may be involved and displaced. Some would regard it wise to note the position and appearance of the kidneys and ureters.

134

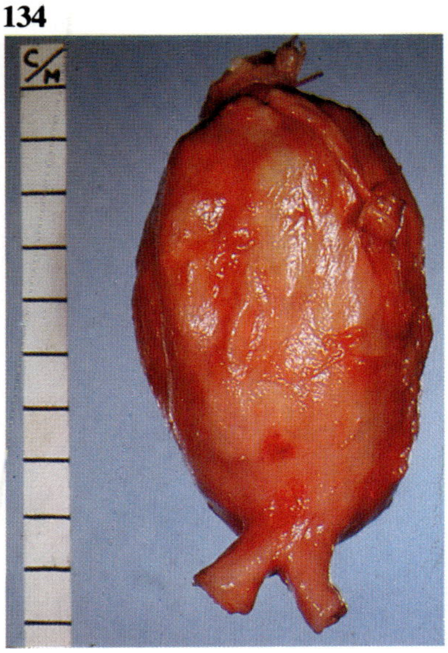

134 A large aneurysm of aorta may, if not ruptured, be excised in toto with the bifurcation of the sac; or it may be opened and the graft laid therein.

135

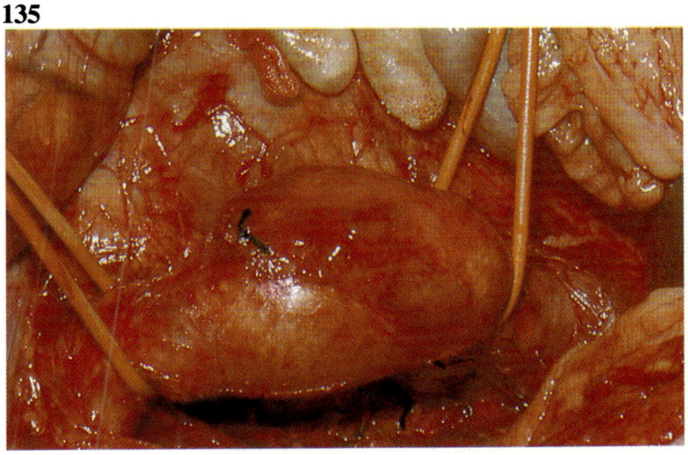

135 Resected aneurysm. This smaller aneurysm was causing a fair amount of abdominal discomfort in an 82-year-old lady who was in good health. Because the risk of rupture increases with the size of the aneurysm and the presence of pain, it was resected. The ligated origin of the inferior mesenteric artery is seen on the aneurysm.

136

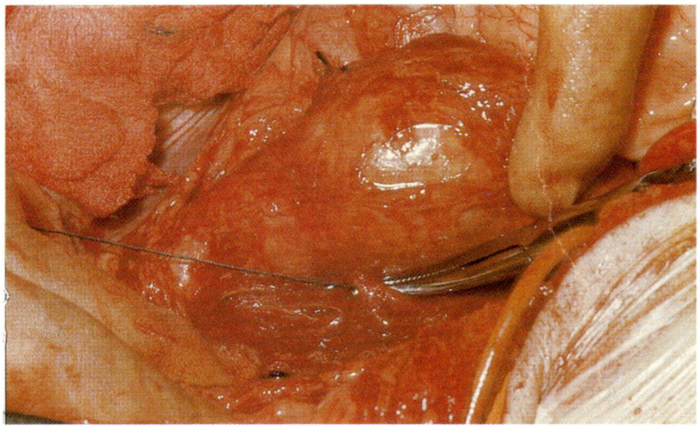

136 Isolation of aneurysm. This required isolation of the aneurysm by clamping below the left renal vein and in this case above the bifurcation. One of the lumbar arteries is shown being islolated and ligated. With all lumbar arteries entering the aneurysm ligated, it was removed.

137

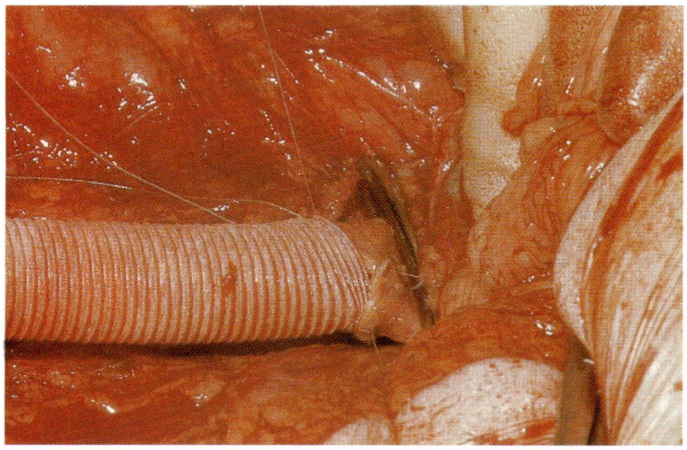

137 The aneurysm is replaced by a graft, in this case made of Dacron, sutured to the aorta below the renal vessels and to the aortic bifurcation.

138

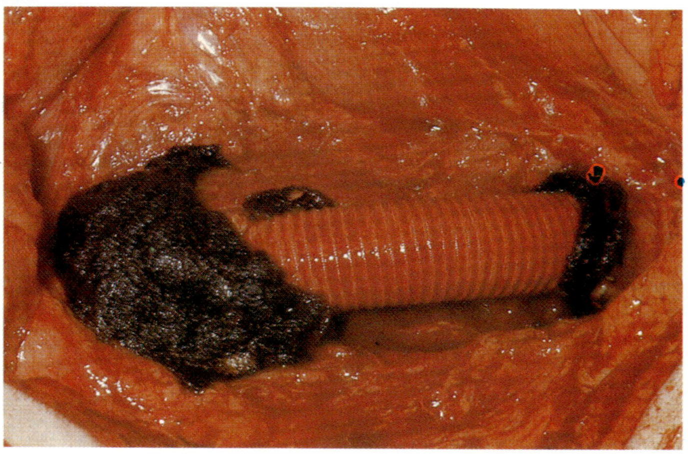

138 The finished operation with graft in situ. The black material is 'Surgicel' which helps to stop the oozing at the anastomotic areas while the heparin is being reversed.

139

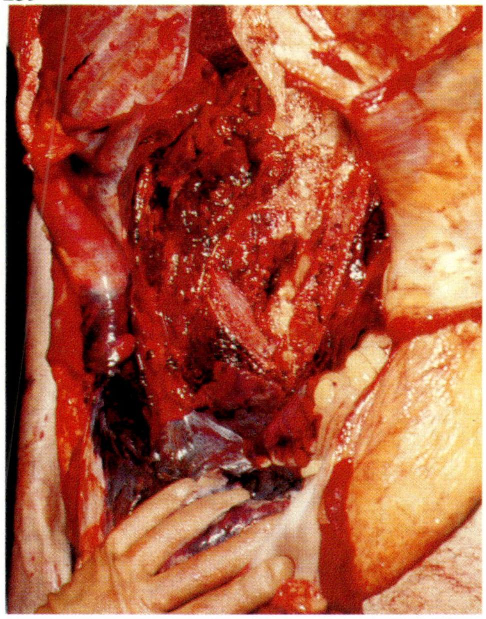

139 Rupture of the aorta is a dreaded complication which occurs with aneurysms greater than 6 cm in diametre and associated with pain. The painful aneurysm should be resected, if at all possible. The aneurysm in this patient had ruptured to the right—the less common side. Death occurred before operation was possible.

140

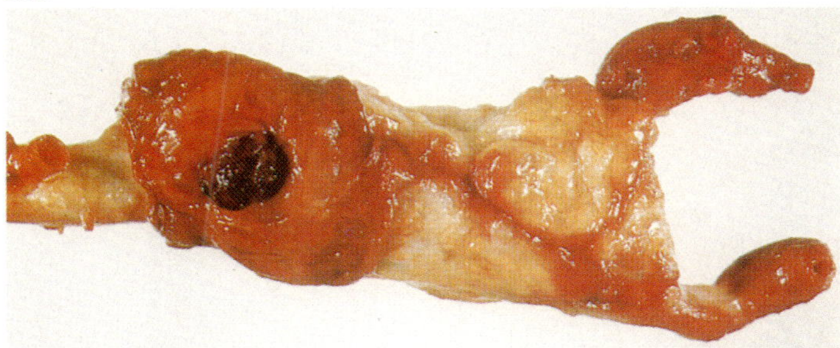

140 Aortoduodenal fistula. A rare type of rupture of an aneurysm is into the duodenum producing an aortoduodenal fistula with haemorrhage and death. Symptoms similar to a peptic ulcer may presage the rupture. The specimen is that of an aortic aneurysm with, in front, a portion of the duodenum containing blood clots.

141

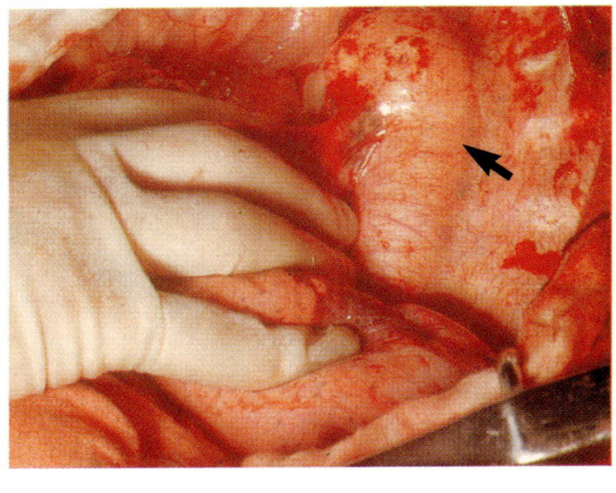

141 Aneurysm of thoracic aorta is often symptomless being picked up on a plain x-ray of chest as an expanded aorta. They may be short and saccular or long and fusiform extending down to diaphragm and below. In this patient, a 57-year-old woman, the aneurysm was short and resectable.

142

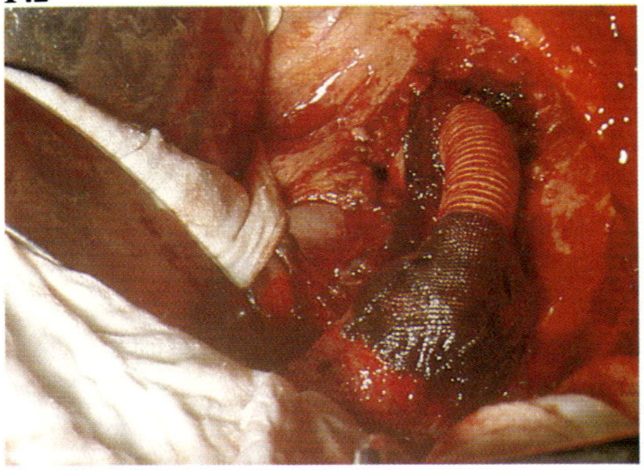

142 Arteriosclerotic aneurysm. The previous aneurysm, which was arteriosclerotic in type, was replaced by a Dacron graft.

143

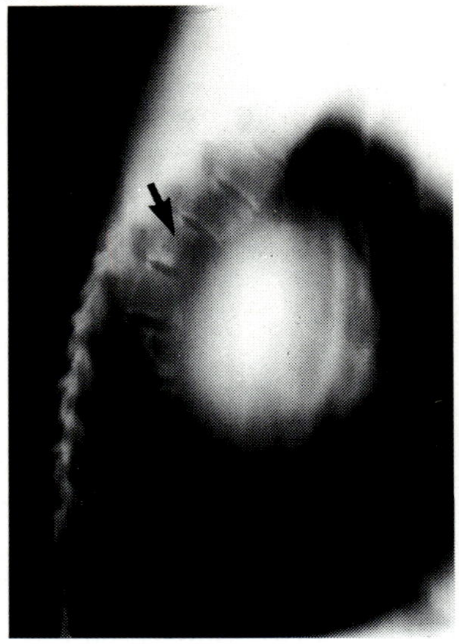

143 Syphilitic aneurysm. Syphilis was once the dominant cause of thoracic aneurysms but they are now less common than those due to ASO. The x-ray shows the erosion of the vertebral bodies caused by a massive syphilitic aneurysm, which are usually saccular.

144

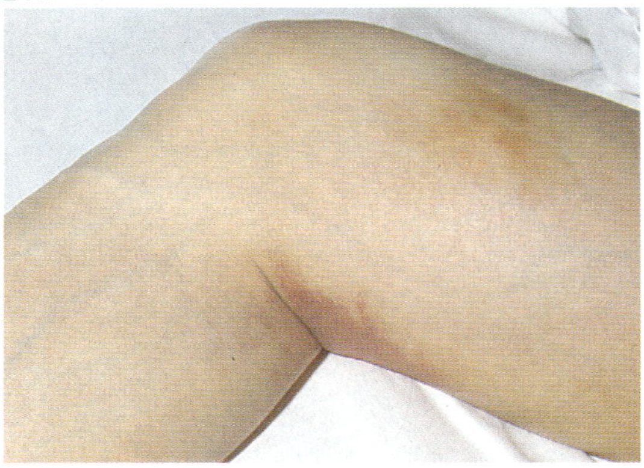

144 Aneurysms of the popliteal artery are not uncommon. They are commonly bilateral and without symptoms until thrombosis, peripheral embolism, or rupture occurs. This patient was aware of a throbbing mass behind the knee. These aneurysms should not be confused with cystic lesions in the popliteal area.

145

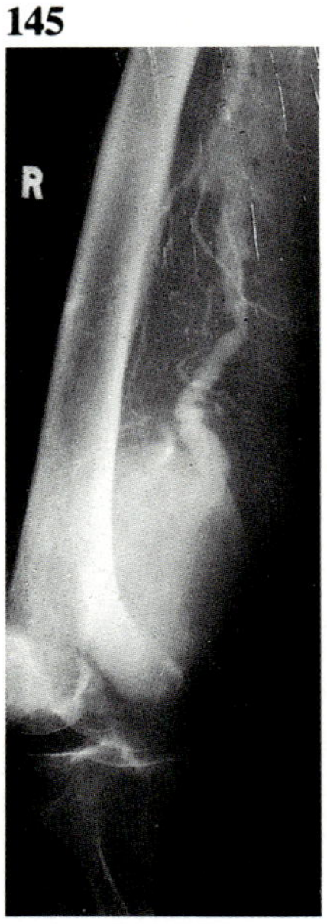

145 Unhealthy artery. Angiography is done not so much to establish diagnosis as to demonstrate the distal arterial tree and allow judgement as to the type of surgery that might be required. The artery above is unhealthy, and no vessels are seen below. The prognosis for limb survival is not good.

146

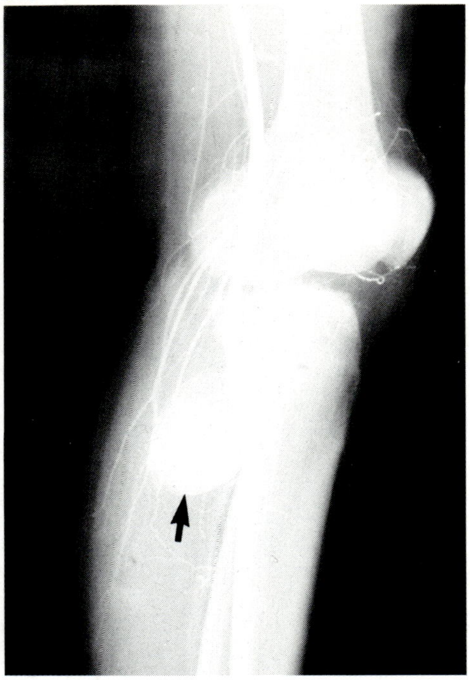

146 **Saccular aneurysm.** This is a small saccular aneurysm which might be amenable to graft replacement except it is near the bifurcation of the artery.

147

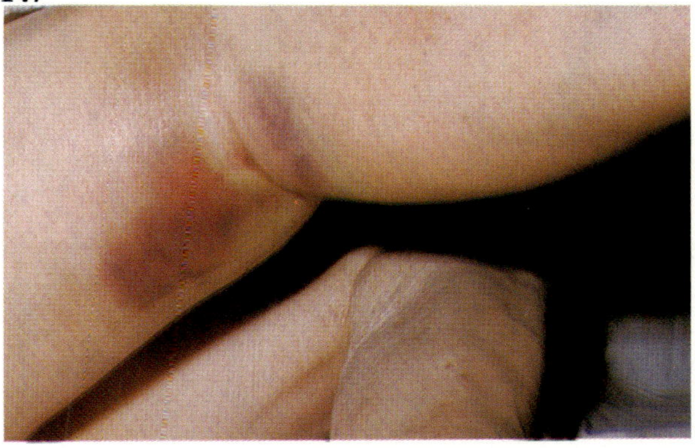

147 **Rupture of a popliteal aneurysm** is indicated by pain and, as in this case, reddening or bruising under the skin. Acute ischaemic changes will occur in the foot.

148

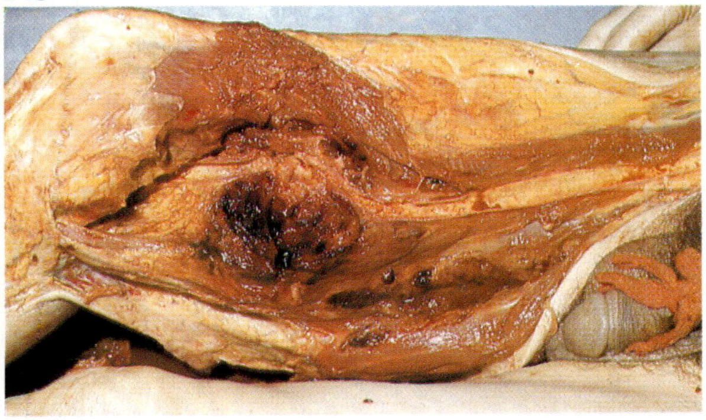

148 **Thrombotic aneurysm.** The above patient died before operation and at post mortem the leak from the thrombotic aneurysm was displayed.

149

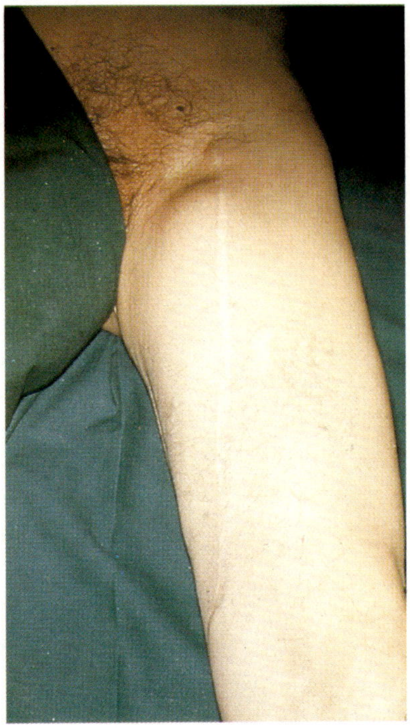

149 **This femoral artery aneurysm** occurred at the site of the insertion of a reversed saphenous vein graft. There was no pain, only a noticeable pulsating swelling.

150

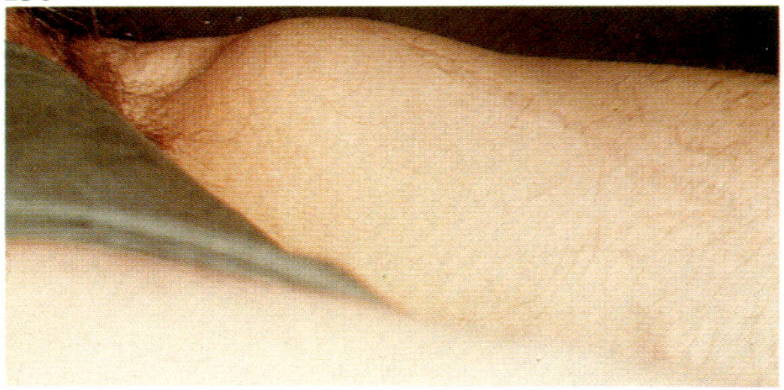

150 Aneurysm size. The lateral view serves to emphasise the size of the aneurysm and its relationship to the previous incision.

151

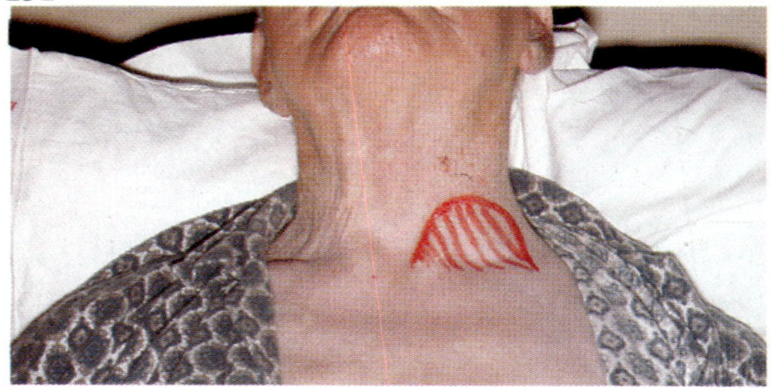

151 A subclavian aneurysm is outlined in the left supraclavicular fossa. A pulsatile mass is easily felt but the patient really had few symptoms. He was merely aware of something different on that side.

152

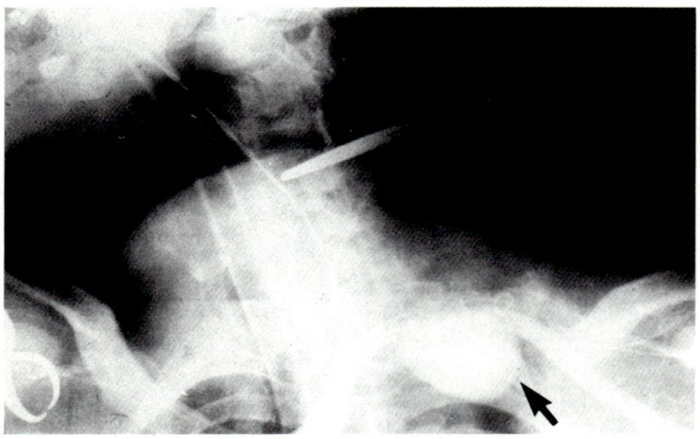

152 Saccular aneurysm. An arteriogram demonstrates an aneurysm which was of the saccular type and due to ASO.

153

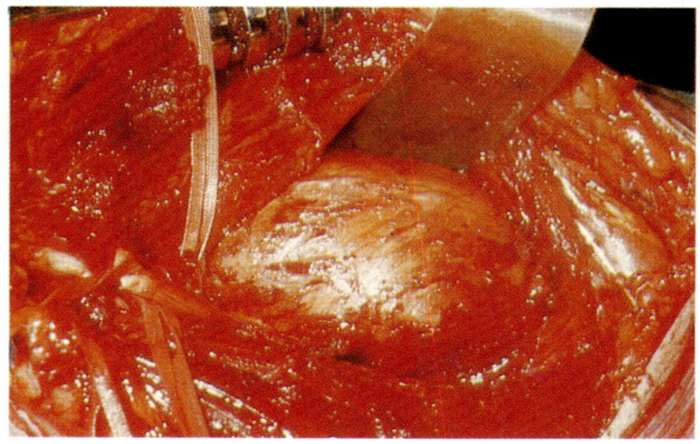

153 Exposure of a subclavian aneurysm. It is not always an easy matter in the large aneurysms to get control of the vessels and avoid damage to the brachial plexus.

154

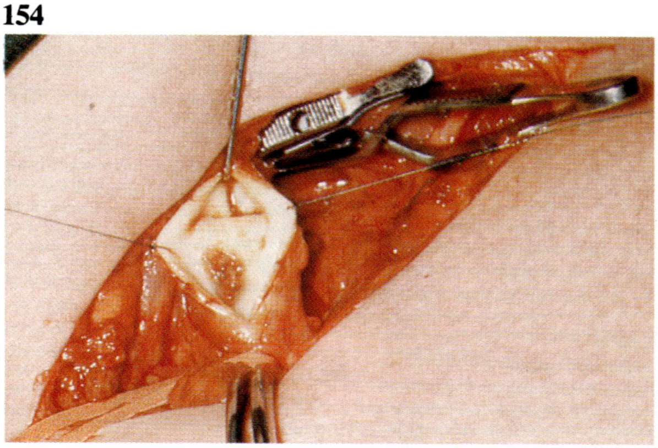

154 This small subclavian aneurysm lay over the top of a cervical rib and when opened up the small thrombus within was seen. Such thrombi could produce distal embolism.

155

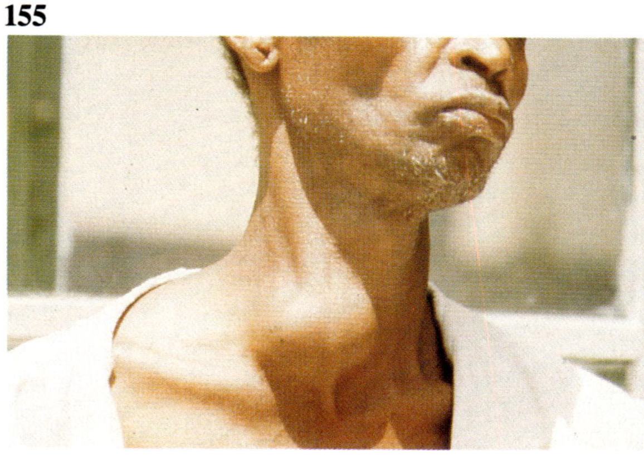

155 This large aneurysm arose from the first part of the subclavian artery. It was syphilitic in origin.

156

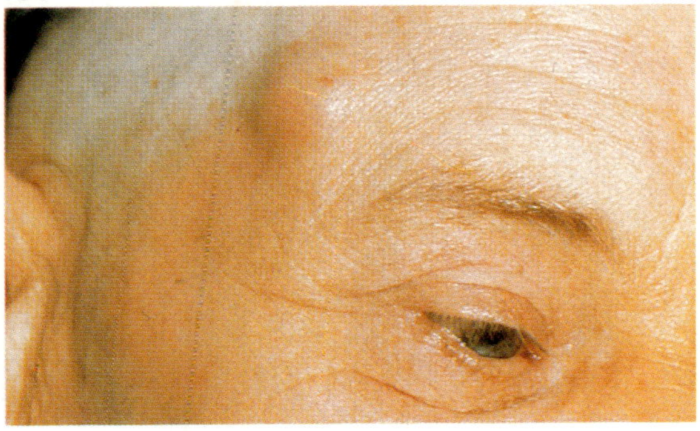

156 Temporal artery aneurysm. This swelling in the right temporal region was a temporal artery aneurysm.

157

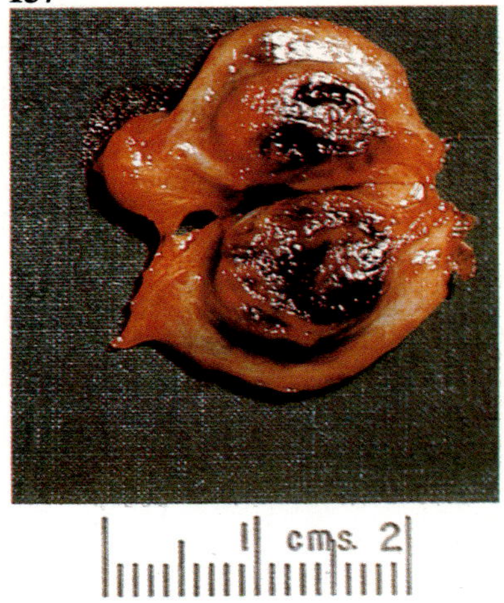

157 Mycotic aneurysm. The excised aneurysm of the temporal artery was found to be a mycotic aneurysm, the result of damage to the wall of the artery by infection—a false aneurysm.

158

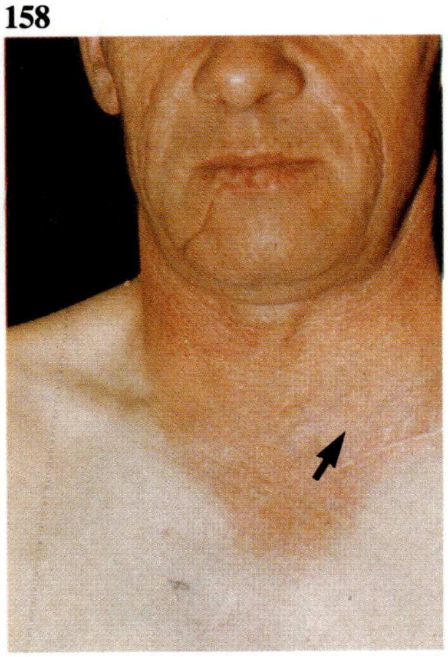

158 Mycotic aneurysm: subclavian artery. A year later the patient reappeared with a further aneurysm, again mycotic, of the left subclavian artery. This is a rare site for this infective type aneurysm.

159

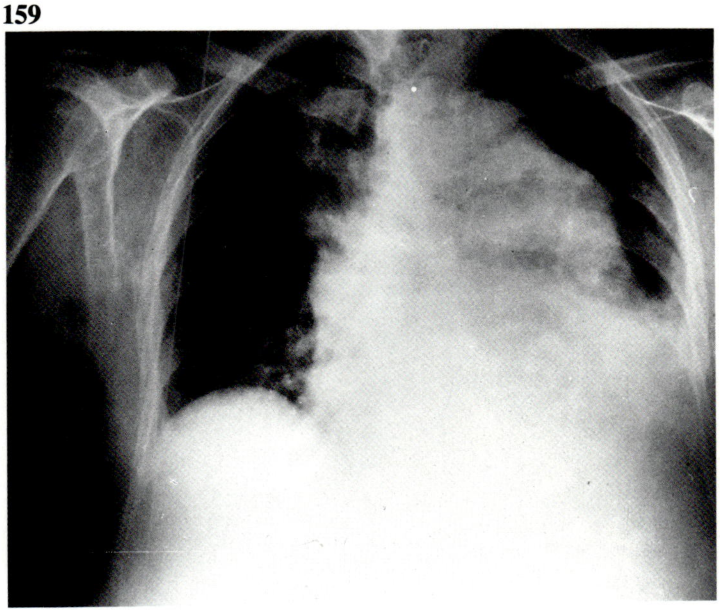

159 A dissecting aneurysm presents with a tearing pain in the back of the thorax passing downwards, shock and dyspnoea. Plain x-ray shows a broadened mediastinum and a fluid (blood) collection in the left chest. Previous hypertension may be a factor.

160

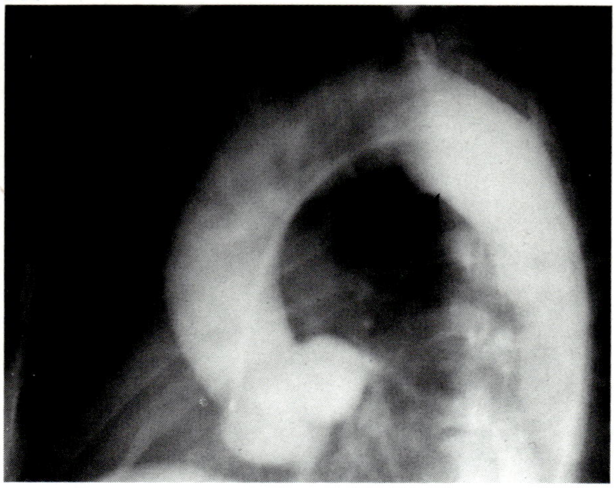

160 Diagnosis of dissecting aneurysm. The diagnosis should be confirmed by aortography which will indicate the origin of the dissection and possibly re-entry. The tear may begin above the aortic valve, ascending aorta and just distal to the origin of the left subclavian artery as shown here. The arrows indicate the double lumen.

161

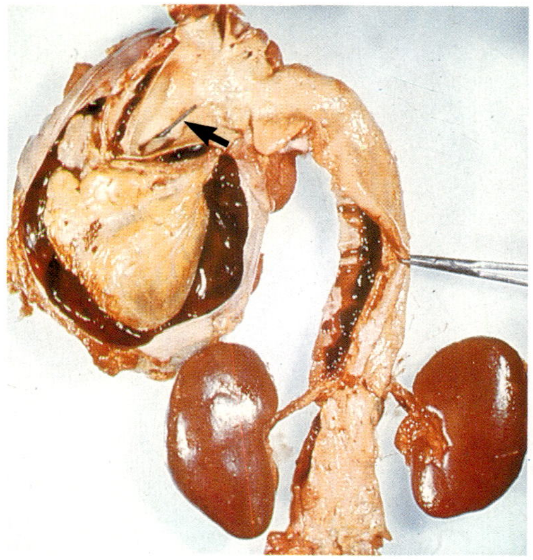

161 Type 1 dissecting aneurysm. This illustrates the type 1 dissection beginning about 2 cm distal to aortic valve and proceeding down into the abdominal aorta and back into the pericardial sac.

162

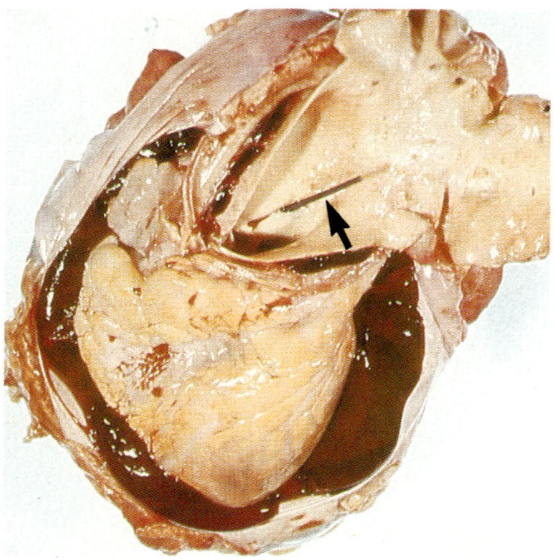

162 Aortic wall tear. The close up demonstrates the tear in the aortic wall, the dissection without the wall and the haemopericardium which, with aortic cusp failure, caused death.

163

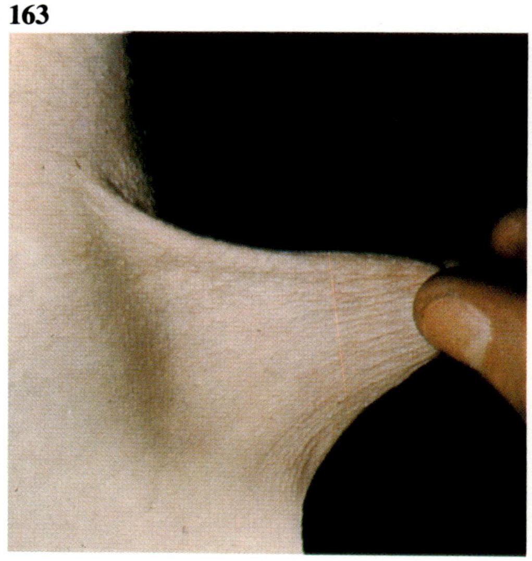

163 Ehlers-Danlos disease, which is a connective tissue disorder that results in loss of elasticity of the tissues, demonstrated here in the skin. Marfan's syndrome is also a known related condition. Both of these may be associated with dissecting aneurysms.

164

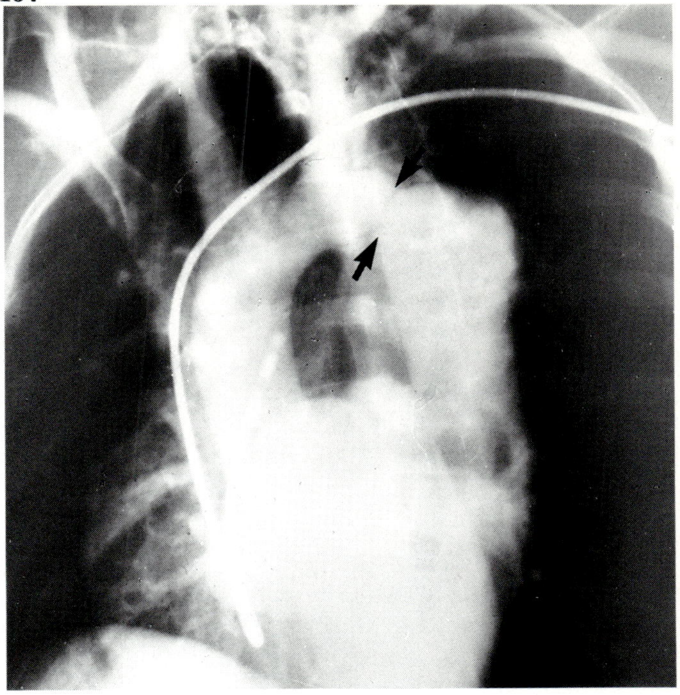

164 A post-stenotic aneurysm may occur beyond a co-arctation of aorta as shown here where the contrast material was injected into the pulmonary artery.

165

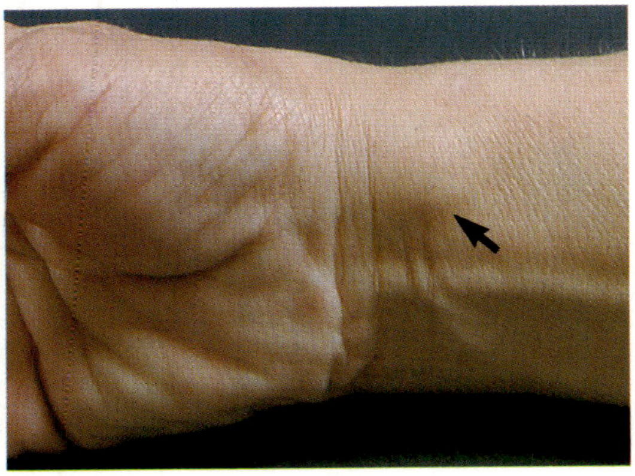

165 Radial artery aneurysm. This patient was referred as a possible aneurysm of the radial artery because of a pulsatile swelling at the wrist. Expansile pulsation was also elicited.

166

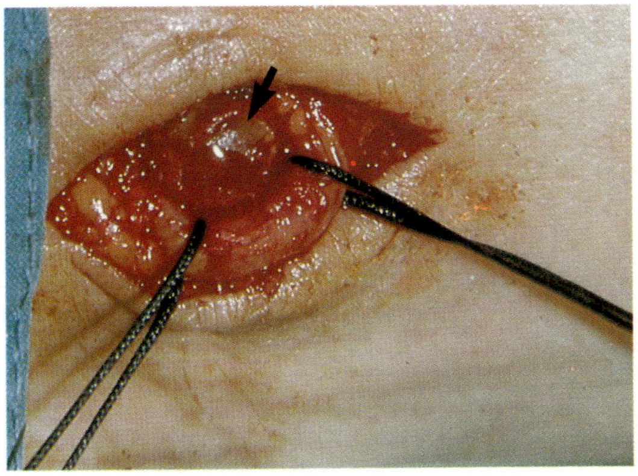

166 Radial artery overlying swelling. A ganglion was diagnosed rather than aneurysm because the swelling would not move from side to side and would not collapse on pressure. This was confirmed at operation. The expansile pulsation was due to a large radial artery overlying the swelling.

6 Vasospastic arterial conditions

Raynaud's syndrome refers to any vasospastic condition where the digital vessels become hypersensitive to changes in temperature. This includes primary Raynaud's syndrome (Raynaud's disease) and secondary Raynaud's syndrome.

Primary Raynaud's syndrome
(Raynaud's Disease)

Criteria
Digits white, blue, red in response to cold
Bilateral or symmetrical
Episodes over two years
No primary cause known
Nutritional changes in skin only

Secondary Raynaud's syndrome

Vascular compression, e.g. cervical rib
Vibration vasospasm
Occlusive arterial disease
Connective tissue disorder, 'vasculitis'
Neurogenic e.g. limb paralysis
Trauma
Drugs: cigarettes
Cold injury
Causalgia

167

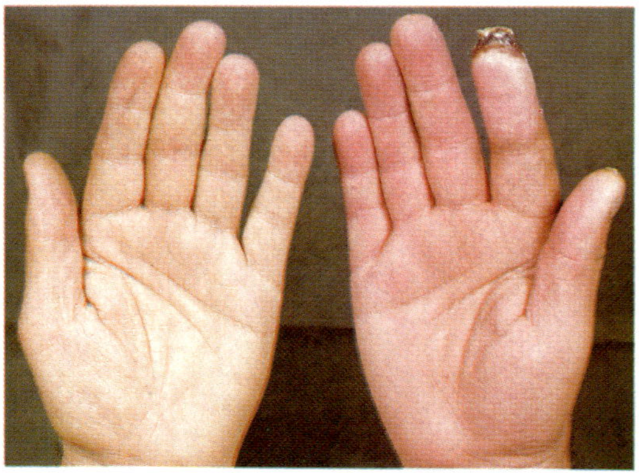

167 In Raynaud's disease there is an idiopathic vasoconstriction of the vessels of the hand in response to cold. The fingers undergo the changes white, blue and finally, on release of vasoconstriction, red. The vasospasm is due to an increased reactivity of the smooth muscle in the blood vessels which are otherwise normal.

168

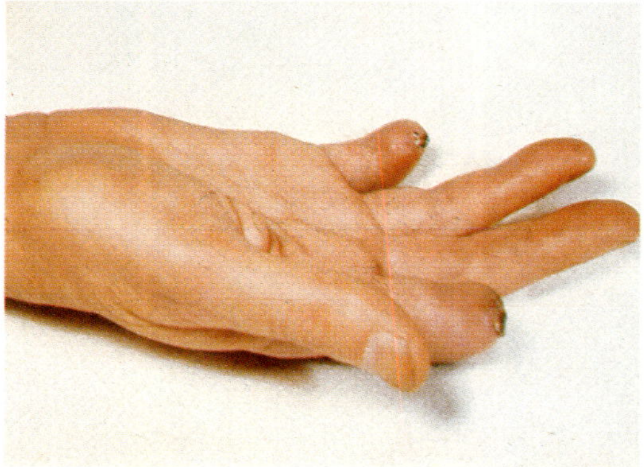

168 Severe Raynaud's disease. In the more severe forms, Raynaud's disease may go on to trophic changes in the fingertips with ulceration and gangrene. Surgical sympathectomy may partially prevent these progressing.

169

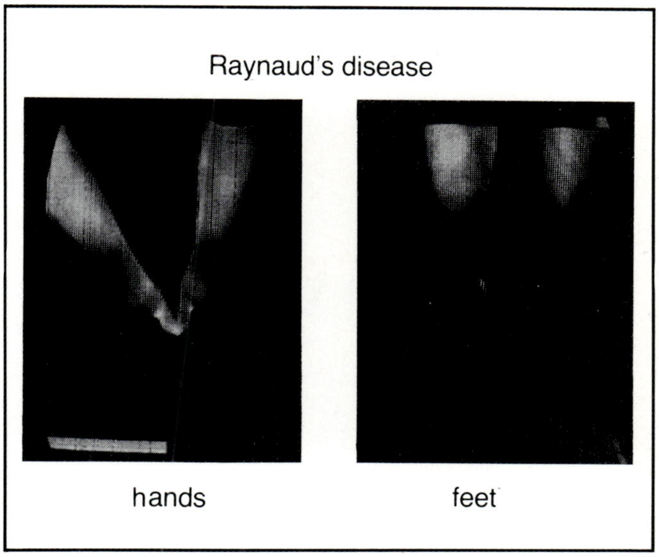

169 Thermography in Raynaud's syndrome will show, during an attack, nearly complete disappearance of the fingers as a result of vasospasm. In this patient the feet were also affected as seen on the right. The white areas are warm and the black areas are cold.

170

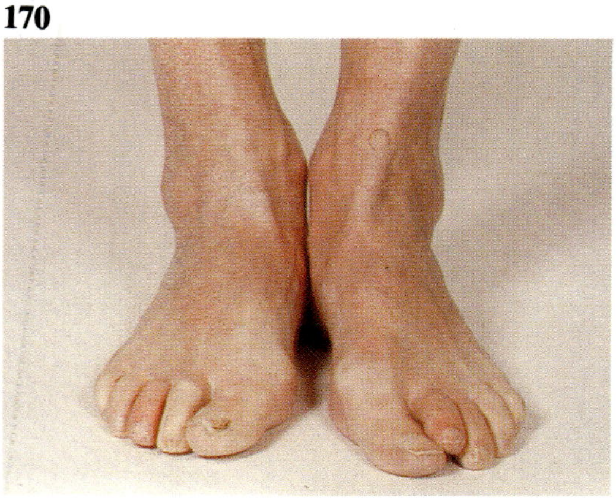

170 Affected toes in Raynaud's syndrome. That the feet may also be affected in Raynaud's disease is shown here where the big toes and some of the others are affected.

171

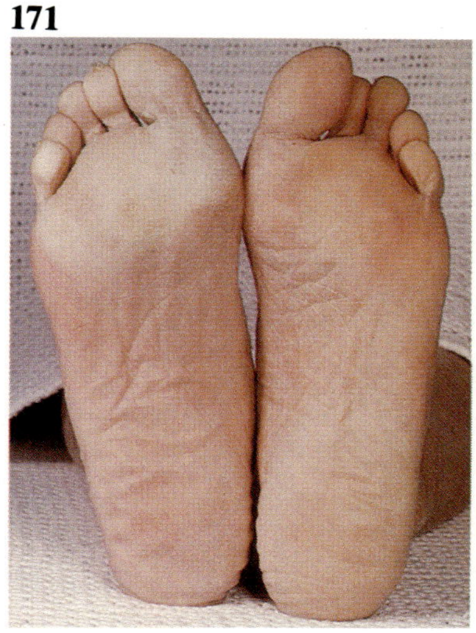

171 Skin pallor in Raynaud's disease. The symmetrical nature of the skin pallor in Raynaud's disease is shown in the soles of the feet and pulps of toes of this individual.

172

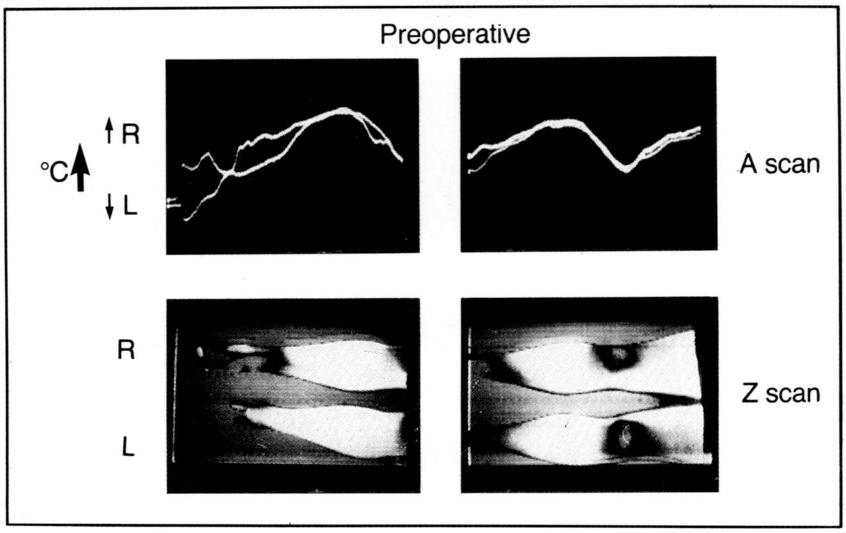

172 Raynaud's disease in legs. On thermoscan of a patient with severe Raynaud's disease in the legs, note the dark areas of poor blood flow. The white areas are warm with good blood flow. The A scan shows the actual temperature changes with a fall at the knees and feet.

173

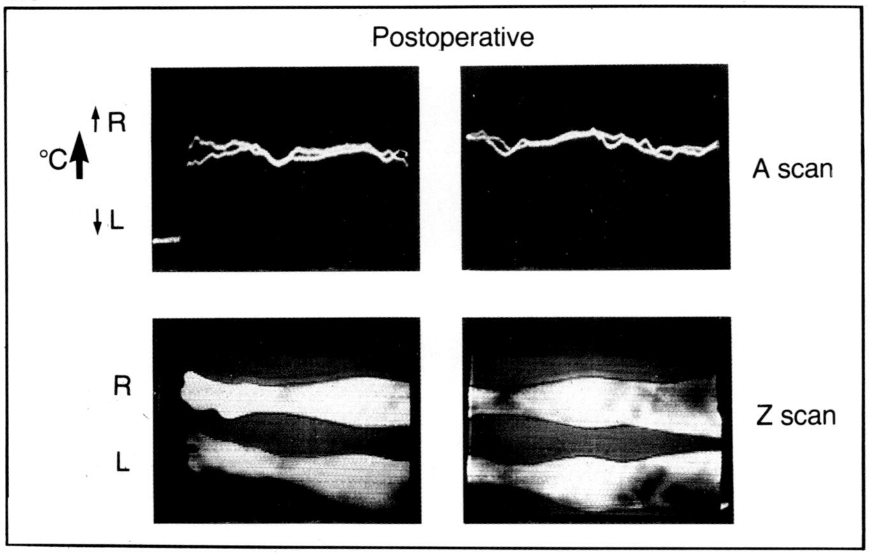

173 Bilateral lumbar sympathectomy. The above patient had a bilateral lumbar sympathectomy with a good effect. The feet became warm. The thermoscan illustrates the recovery of skin blood flow by an increase in the white area.

174

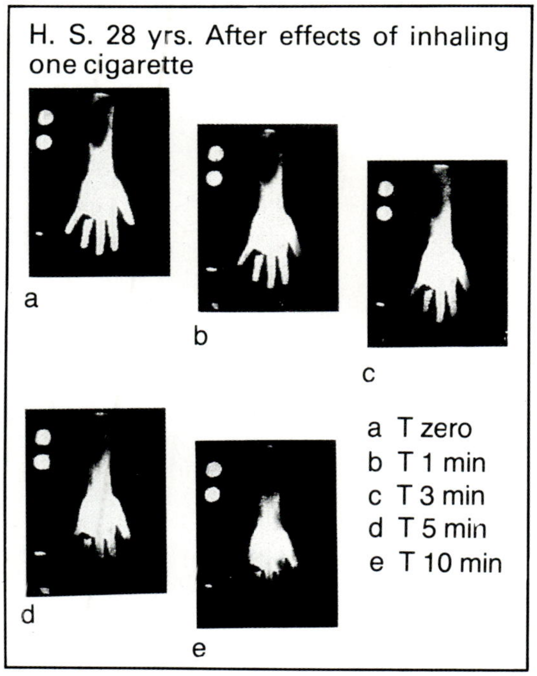

174 Diminution in skin blood flow. The effect of drugs can be seen in some normal individual after smoking cigarettes. The gradual disappearance of the finger with time indicates a diminution in skin blood flow. No one with Raynaud's phenomenon should smoke.

175

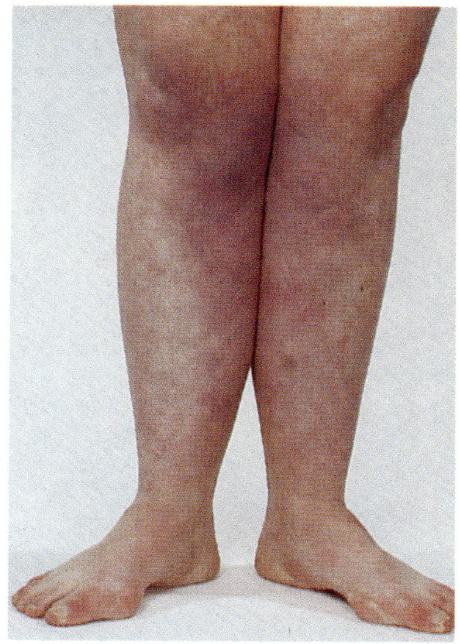

175 **Acrocyanosis** is not really a form of Raynaud's syndrome; it is a vasoconstrictive disorder appearing in young females where a cyanotic appearance is present in hands and feet. The limbs are cold and, as here, the cyanosis may have a reticulated pattern, the so-called livedo reticularis. Warm clothing will help with sympathectomy reserved for the severe cases.

176

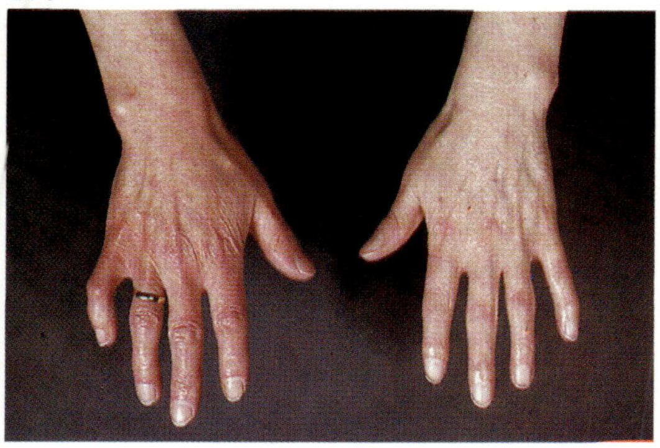

176 Secondary Raynaud's phenomenon. Unilateral vasospasm suggests a secondary Raynaud's phenomenon with an underlying cause which should be looked for. In this patient, with post-traumatic vasomotor dystrophy, it affected the left hand.

177

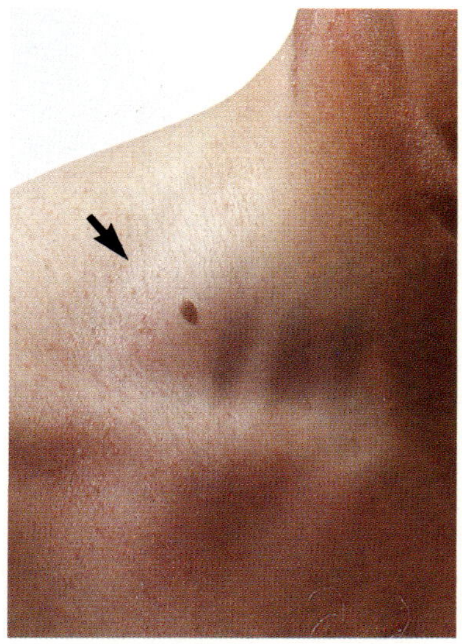

177 Unilateral Raynaud's syndrome. A not infrequent cause of unilateral Raynaud's syndrome is a cervical rib which may produce visible evidence by filling up the supracalvicular fossa. The left fossa was less prominent than the right.

178

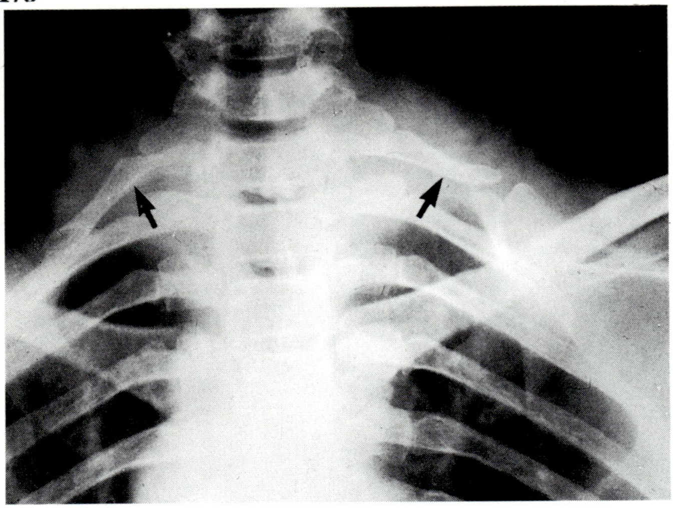

178 Bilateral cervical ribs. Plain x-ray of the neck showed bilateral cervical ribs, the one on the left side being more prominent than that on the right.

179

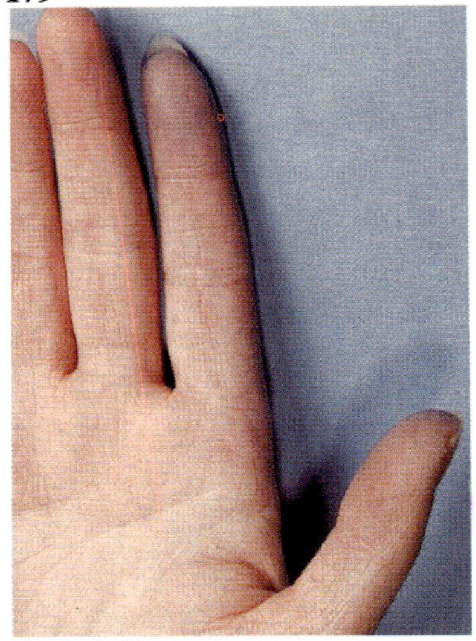

179 Vasospastic response in fingers. The patient may present with tingling and numbness usually of inner border of the hand but sometimes a vasospastic type of response is seen in the fingers, particularly the index. In this case the index finger felt cold and a slight bluish tinge was seen in the pulp of the finger.

180

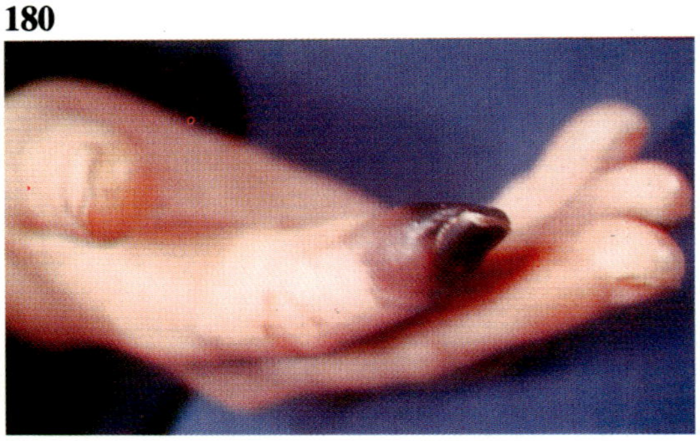

180 The digital ischaemia with gangrene was due to emboli arising from the artery just distal to the cervical rib. An arteriogram will show a lesion in the subclavian artery.

181

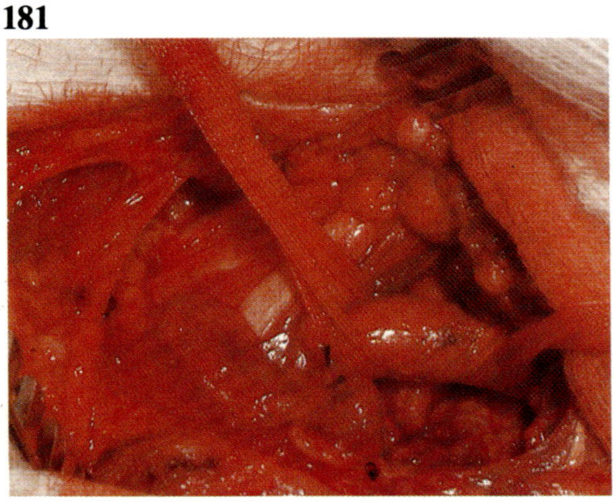

181 The subclavian artery is shown between the tapes overlying a cervical rib. The distal portion of the artery is a little dilated as it passes over and beyond the rib.

182

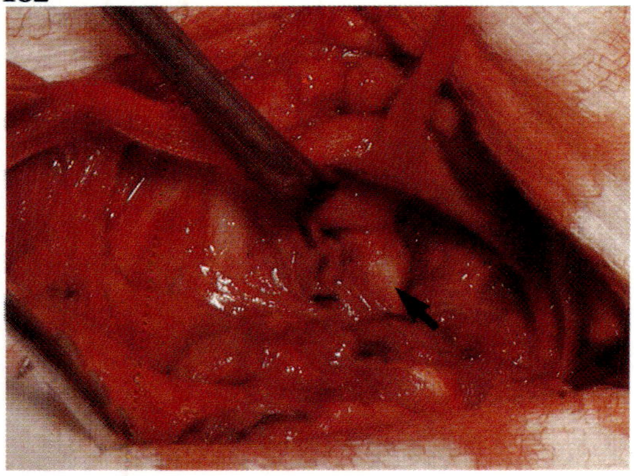

182 Elevated subclavian artery. With the artery elevated the cervical rib is more easily seen.

183

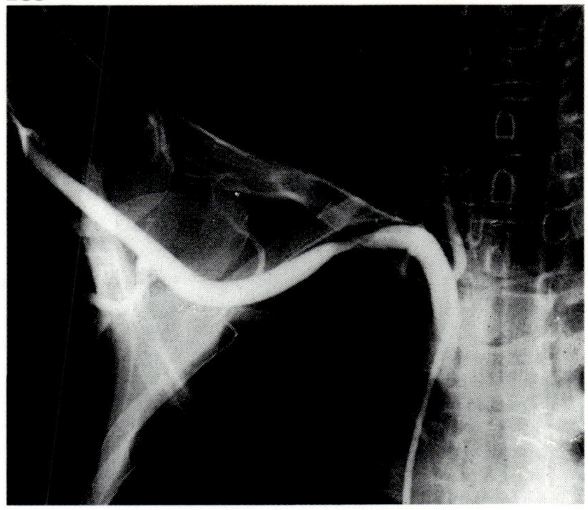

183 Narrowing of the subclavian artery may also be due to throacic outlet compression, in this case thought to be due to pressure of muscles as the arm is hyperabducted.

Vibration tool disease

184

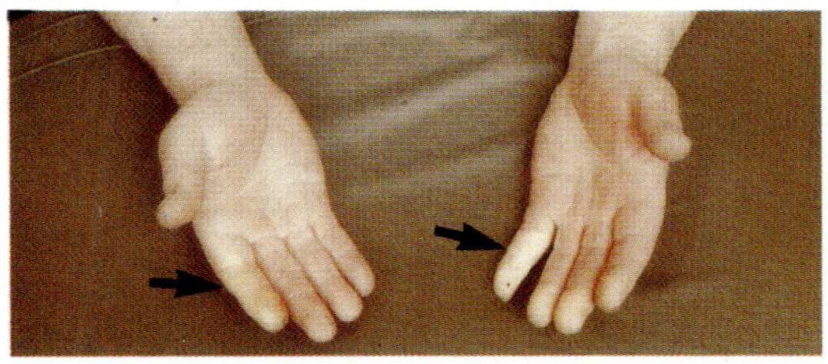

184 Power-saw induced vasospasm. The cause of this patient's vasospasm was the continual use of a power saw. His symptoms appeared within one year of starting work.

185

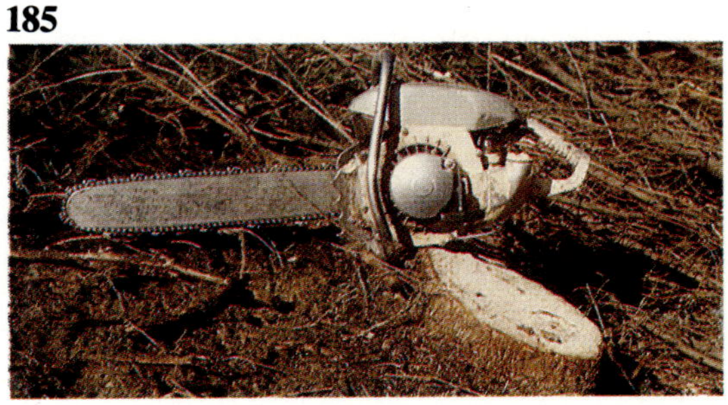

185 The power saw is only one of a variety of tools giving this condition the name 'vibration tool disease'. It usually occurs after some years exposure. Other tools include hand grinding tools, pneumatic stone cutters, and mechanical chisels.

186

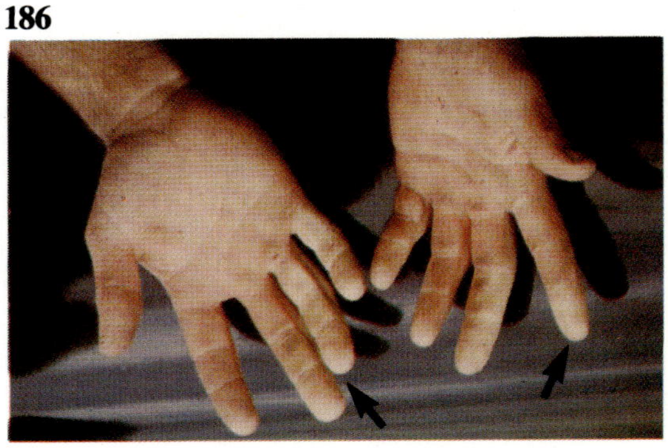

186 Pallor in vibration tool disease. The characteristic pallor seen in the fingers of this patient relate to the way he grips the tool. These fingers which grip strongly are more affected by the vibrations which are at the higher range.

187

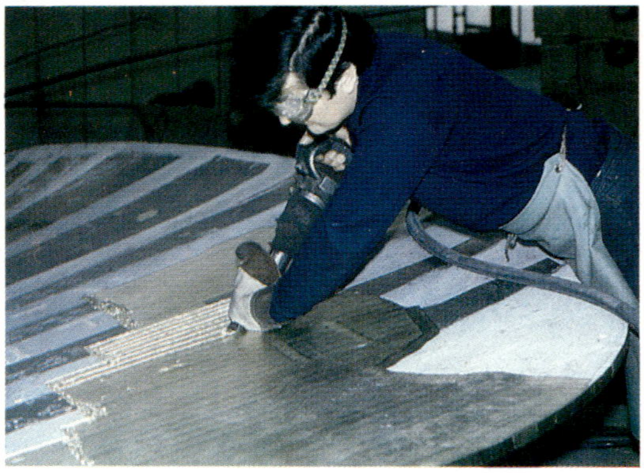

187 Spasms of digital vessels. The above patient gripped the handle of this pneumatic tool with his right hand and the shaft lay in his left hand. The vibration can produce initially spasms of the digital vessels and later thrombosis.

188

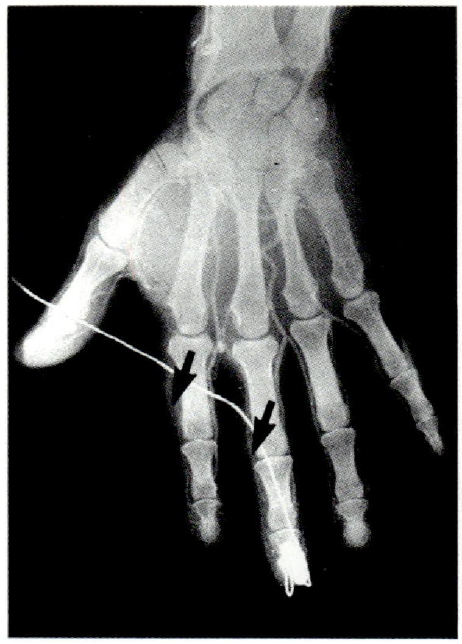

188 Digital artery blocks. Arteriography in these patients may show digital artery blocks, probably the result of platelets adhering to vascular endothelium damaged by the vibrations. A temperature measuring device is attached to the middle finger.

Other causes of secondary Raynaud's syndrome

189

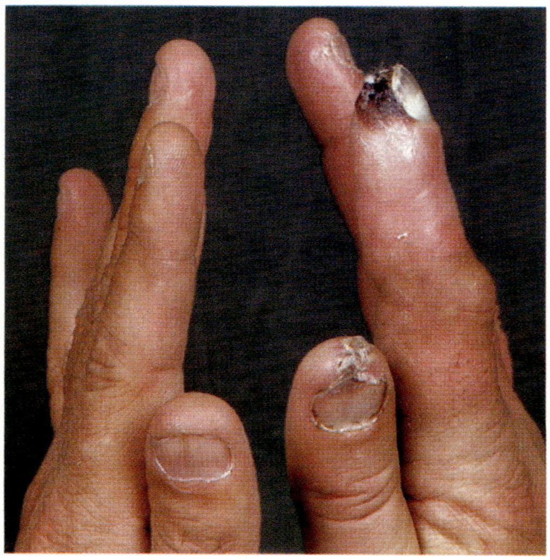

189 Gangrene of fingertip. Raynaud's syndrome may be seen in patients, usually middle-aged males, who have digital artery thrombosis sometimes associated with diabetes. The affected digit may appear normal when warm but on exposure to cold becomes blue, pallor is not so common, and finally as in this case, gangrene of the fingertip may occur.

190

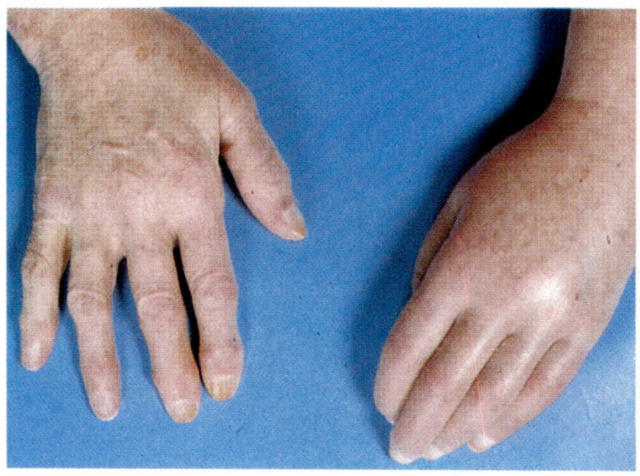

190 Causalgia is associated with vasomotor changes in response to cold. The patient's left hand is swollen, the skin shiny. The burning pain is characteristic. The condition follows injury to the nerves in the upper limb. Sympathectomy, although usually successful, was only so for a short time in this case.

191

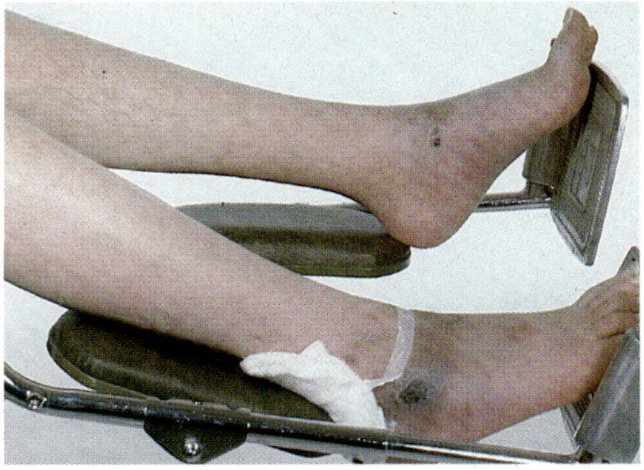

191 Post-traumatic vascular dystrophy. Paralysis of the limbs, as in poliomyelitis or injury, may result in chronic vasoconstriction where the extremities are bluish, cold, and may develop ulcers as shown here in the pressure points round the ankles. This patient had a traumatic paraplegia—the vascular condition may be termed post-traumatic vascular dystrophy. Sympathectomy has a variable response.

Secondary Raynaud's syndrome due to collagen disorders

The collagen disorders are the result of immunological reactions. The exact pathogenesis is not completely clear but it is probable that the connective tissue changes are the result of a vasculitis. This varies with the type of collagen disorder.

192

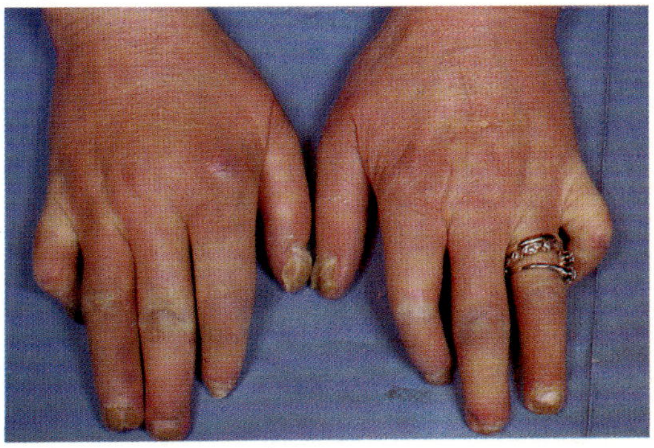

192 Secondary Raynaud's syndrome. This patient was thought for years to have Raynaud's disease but gradually tissue necrosis of the pulps took place. The final diagnosis was secondary Raynaud's syndrome due to scleroderma.

193

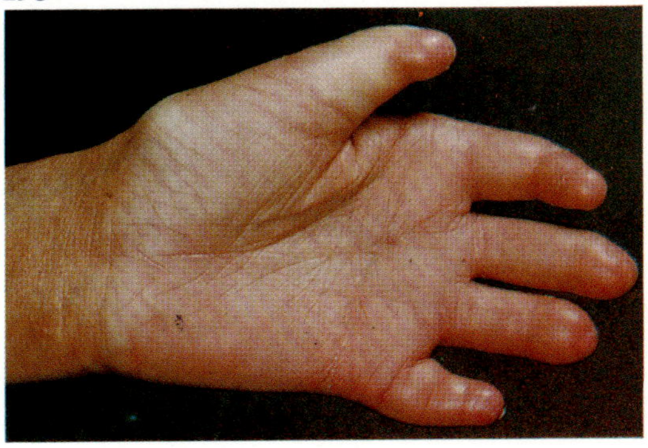

193 The classical skin changes of scleroderma are illustrated: inelasticity, oedema, dermal atrophy and smooth waxy appearance. It usually occurs in women and is associated with Raynaud's syndrome. Calcifications, Raynaud's syndrome, scleroderma and telangiectasia may exist in the CRST syndrome of Winterbauer.

194

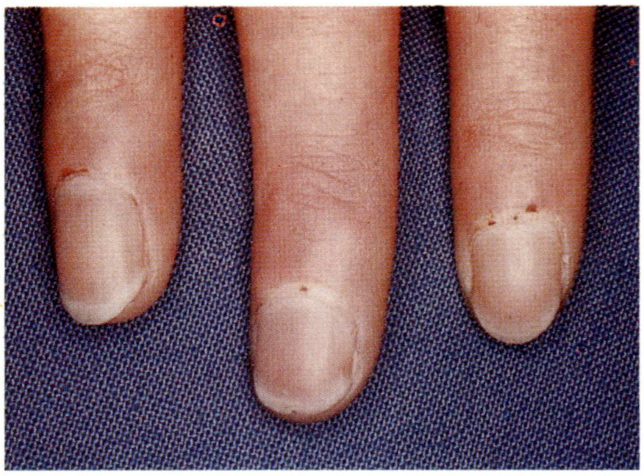

194 Disseminated lupus erythematosus (DLE) is common in women in whom widespread necrosis of small vessels may lead to digital necrosis and gangrene. Splinter haemorrhage in the nailfold indicate a vasculitis. A positive LE cell phenomenon, raised gamma globulin and leucopaenia help to establish the diagnosis.

195

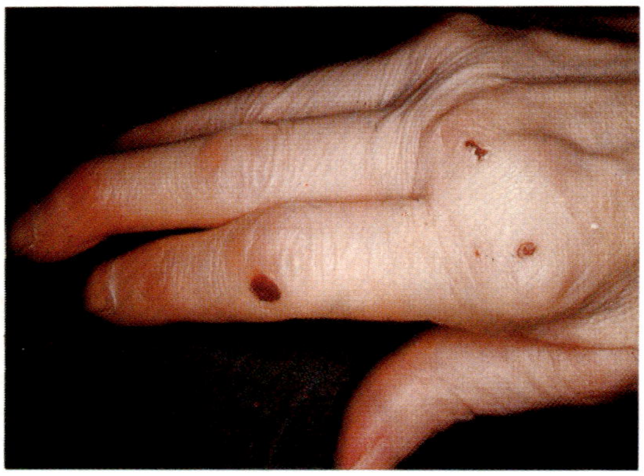

195 In rheumatoid arthritis (RA) intimal hyperplasia may occur affecting small vessels such as those of the digits. Occlusion of these vessels produces dermal infarcts seen in the nailfolds, finger pulps and skin of the hand. The typical joint changes are notable.

196

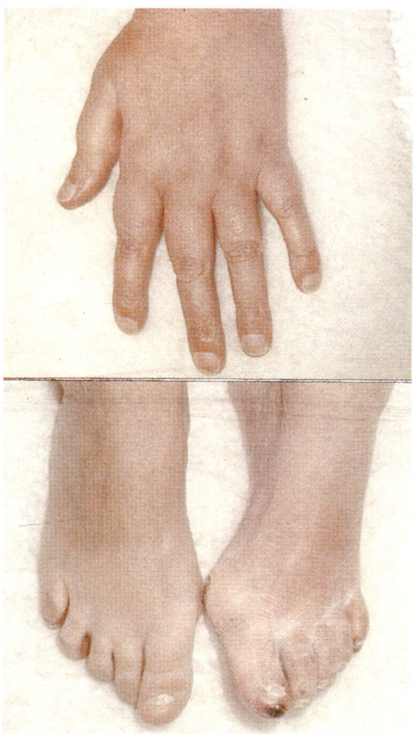

196 Relationship of joints in RA. The combination of RA joints in the hands and the dermal infarcts in the toes, as shown in this composite picture, is highly suggestive of a relationship.

197

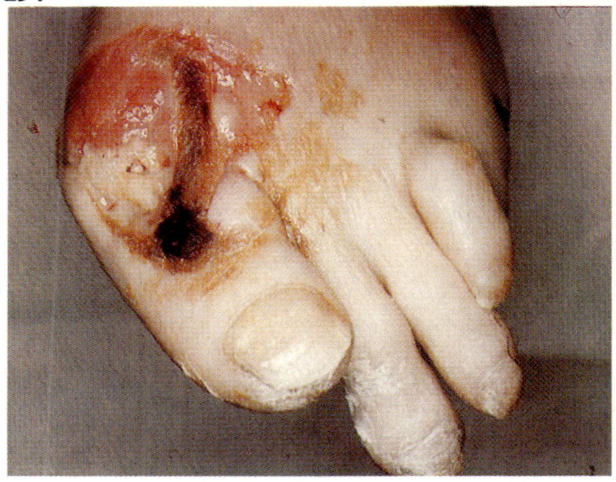

197 Ulceration and peripheral neuropathy in RA. If the RA vasculitis is severe and widespread the dermal infarction may lead to ulceration and a peripheral neuropathy may be present.

198

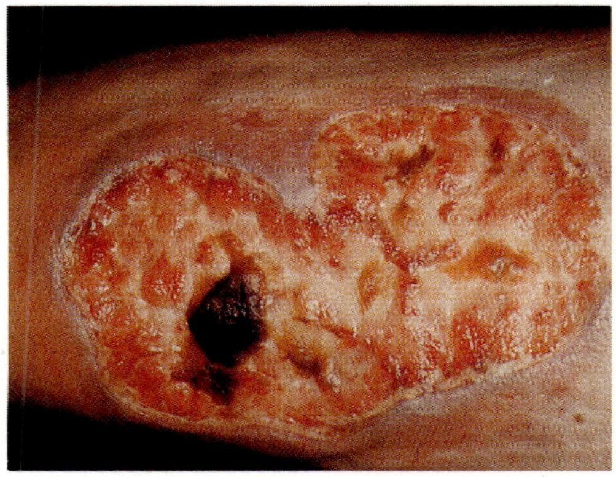

198 Rheumatoid vasculitis. This patient had leg ulcers for nine years. These were thought to be varicose although no varicose veins were present. The association of RA joints and finally biopsy of the lesion established a rheumatoid vasculitis.

199

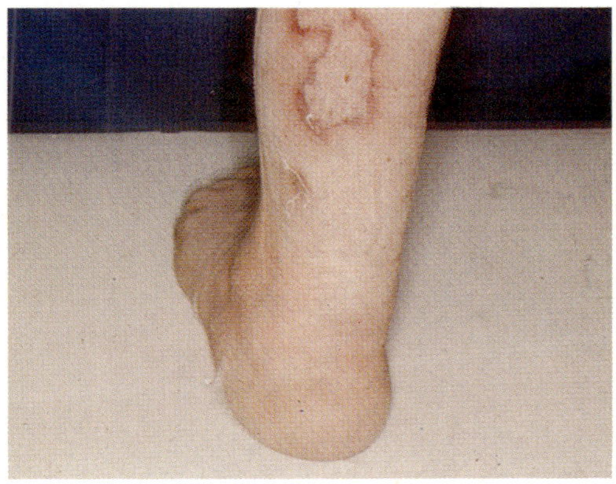

199 Varicose ulcers. The situation of these ulcers is not typical of varicose ulcers. Normal pulses were present. The patient had RA joints with a positive rheumatoid factor.

200

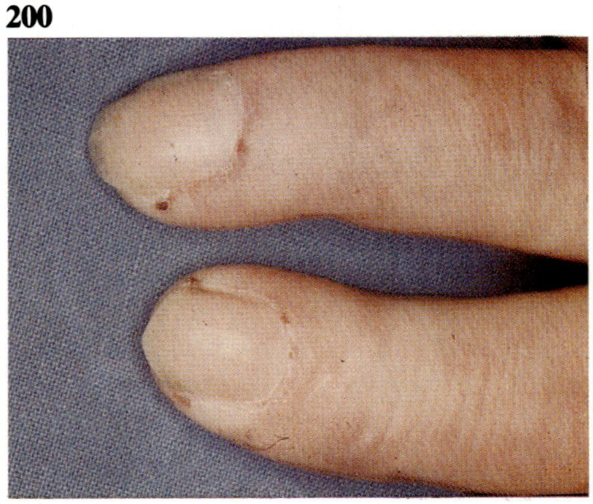

200 Polyarteritis nodosa is another cause of widespread vasculitis. The clinical features are as in other causes of vasculitis. Haemorrhages may be seen in fingers but digital ischaemia is uncommon. The splinter haemorrhages are shown here in the nail folds.

201

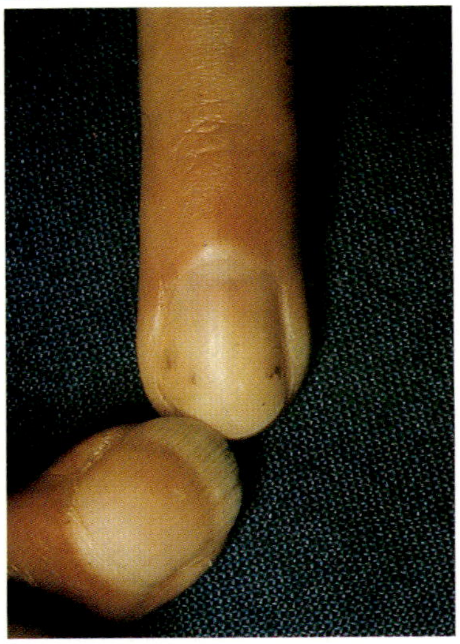

201 The splinter haemorrhages of polyarteritis nodosa are also to be seen in the nails themselves.

202

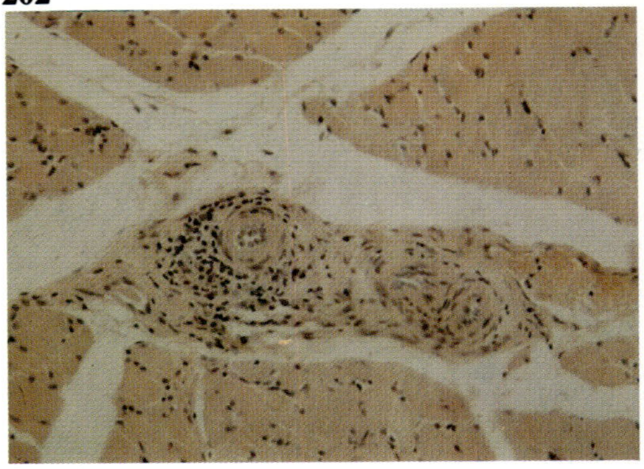

202 Inflamed arteries and arterioles. A biopsy, in this case of muscle, will show the typical inflammatory infiltration of the arteries and arterioles.

203

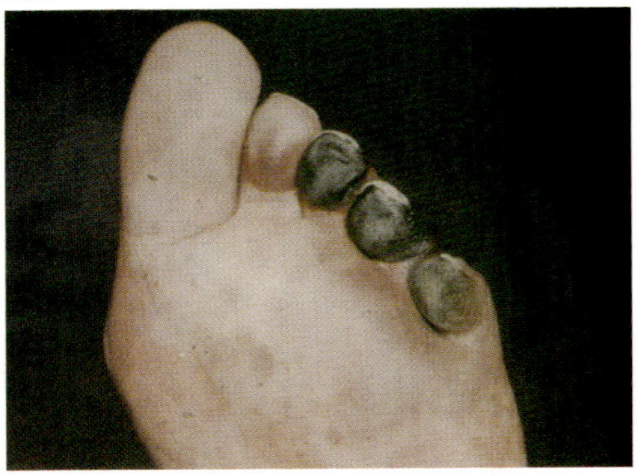

203 Digital ischaemia is not common in polyarteritis nodosa, but it did occur in this patient who also had the splinter haemorrhages in the fingers illustrated above.

204

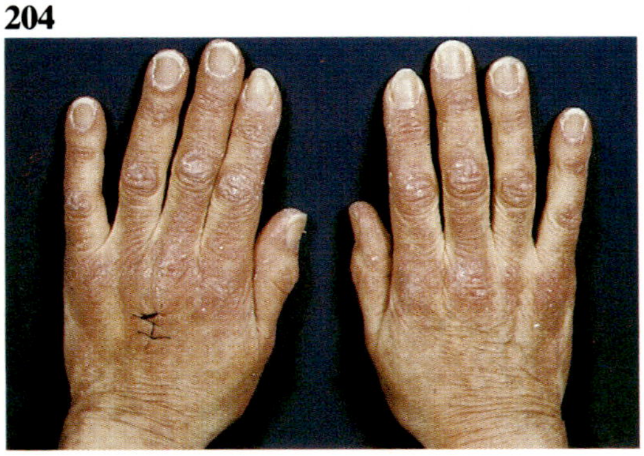

204 Dermatomyositis is an uncommon condition but when it occurs is often accompanied by Raynaud's syndrome. The red colouration of the hands is evident and was associated with fever and a myopathy. Biopsy was done to establish diagnosis.

205

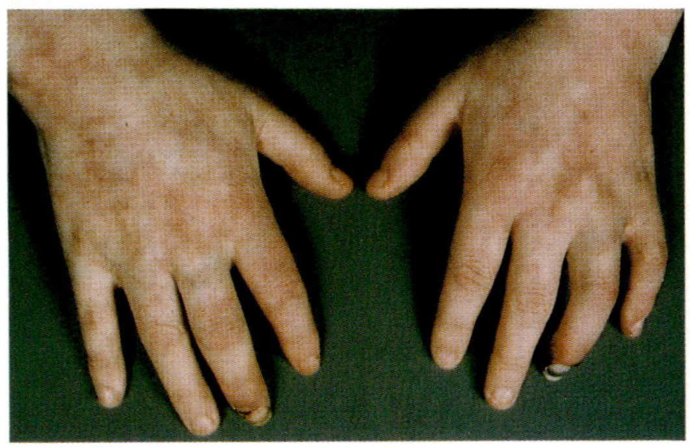

205 Raynaud's phenomenon. The hands are those of a 28-year-old girl who for years had Raynaud's phenomenon with a curious mottled appearance of the skin. The upper limb pulses were absent, 'pulseless disease'.

206

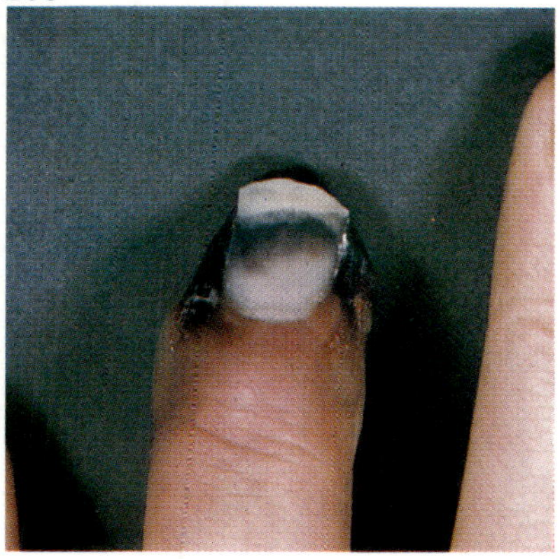

206 Gangrene of the fingertip developed, going on to larger areas of necrosis with pain. Partial amputation and bilateral cervical sympathectomy gave some relief. Incidentally, she was a heavy smoker and could not give it up.

207

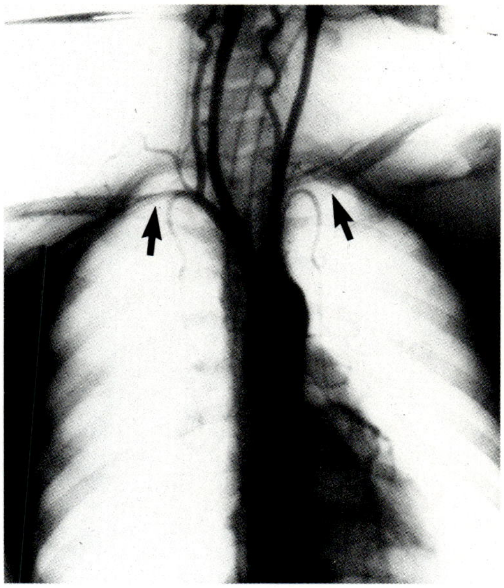

207 Takayasu's disease. Aortogram showed a block in the left subclavian artery and narrowing of the right. This, in a young woman, is typical of the aortic arch syndrome (Takayasu's disease). This is most likely a mixed bag of arterial pathology which is also termed juvenile occlusive aortitis (JOA).

208

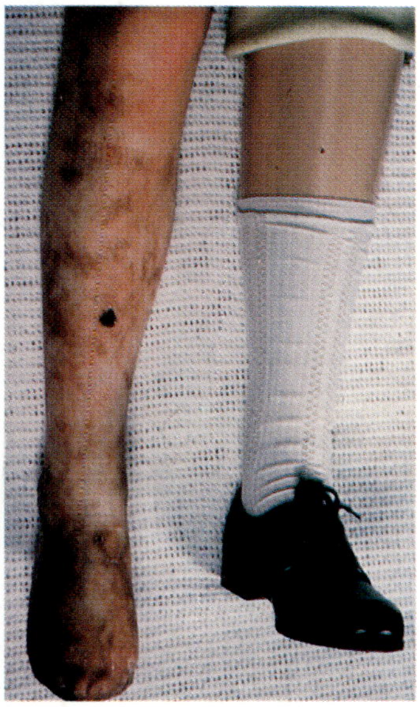

208 Takayasu's disease. The peculiar nature of the disease is emphasised here. The girl already described started to have trouble at 15 years of age, with blockage of a femoral artery requiring amputation. The curious patchy changes in the right leg fit in with an arteritis of unknown origin. Histology was unhelpful as to exact classification.

209

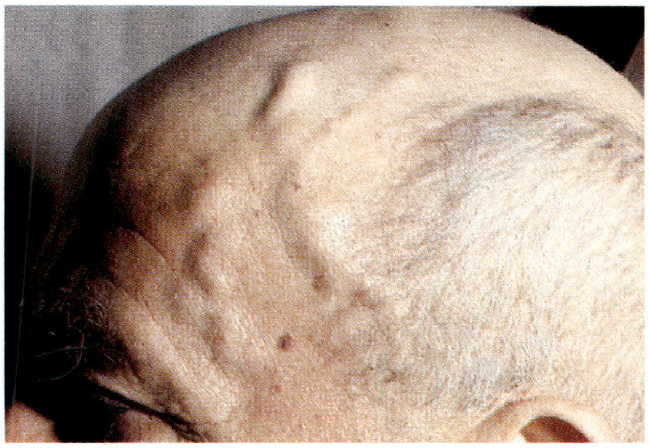

209 Giant cell arteritis is usually easily recognised in the temporal artery (temporal arteritis) where it produces a severe throbbing pain usually in the elderly. The artery is hyperpulsatile and usually evidently so, as here.

210

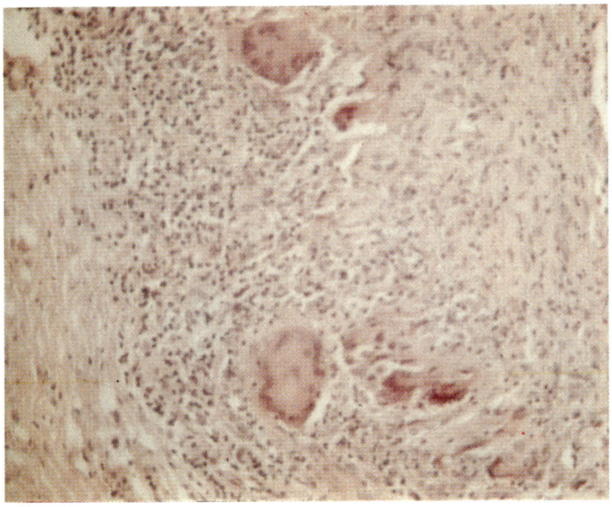

210 Diagnosis by biopsy. Biopsy will confirm the diagnosis. Multinuclear giant cells in this area are diagnostic. Other cells include macrophages and mononuclear cells such as lymphocytes.

211

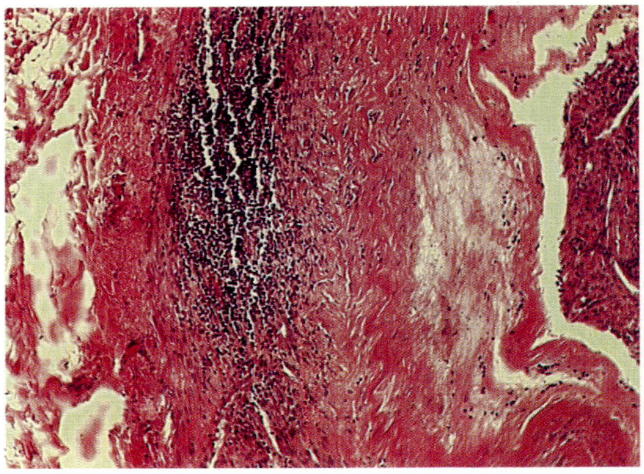

211 Buerger's disease (thromboangiitis obliterans: TAO) can be regarded as a peculiar form of arteritis which occurs almost exclusively in young males who are heavy smokers. This patient smoked 50 cigarettes a day. A migratory thrombophlebitis is often present in such cases. It is not common in the upper limbs.

212

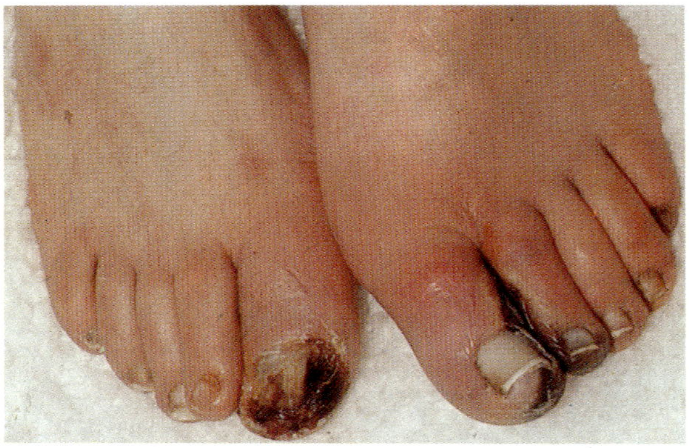

212 Pain and gangrene. This patient presented with pain in both feet and gangrene in the toes. He was 40 years of age. The popliteal pulses were palpable.

213

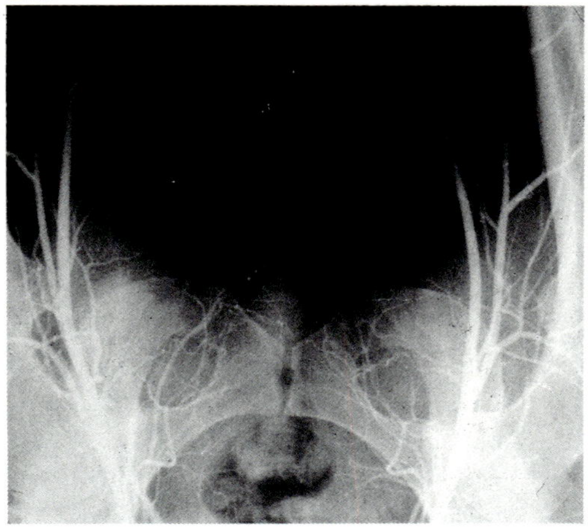

213 Relation between ASO and Buerger's disease. Aortogram was normal until the lower part of the superficial femoral arteries which showed a smooth narrowing in a tapering fashion. This emphasises the link up of arteriosclerosis obliterans and Buerger's disease as they nearly always coexist. Histology of resected toes confirmed the presence of an arteritis.

Cold injury

The effect of cold on the limbs is a combination of vasoconstriction, diminished blood flow, arterial endothelial damage, crystallisation, capillary damage and direct injury to the tissues themselves.

214

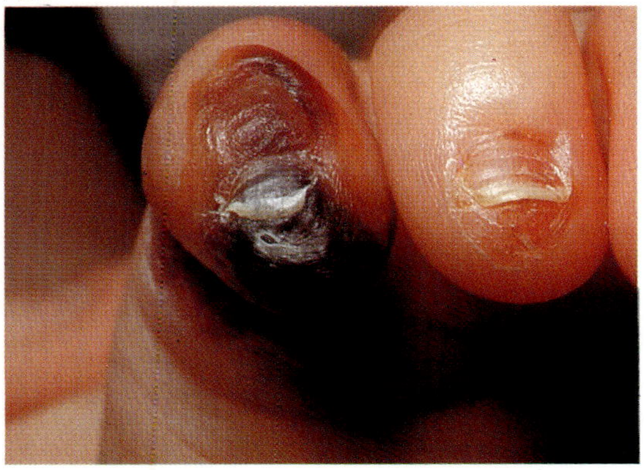

214 Vasospastic changes with damage to the digits may be seen in response to cold—cold injury. The toes in this child's foot were exposed to cold due to defective socks the ends of which were worn off, exposing the tips of the toes to cold.

215

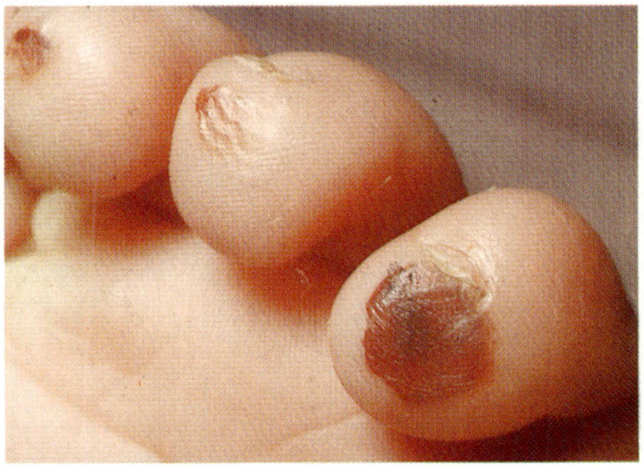

215 Cold injury to toes. The toes of the other foot were similarly but less severely affected by the cold.

216

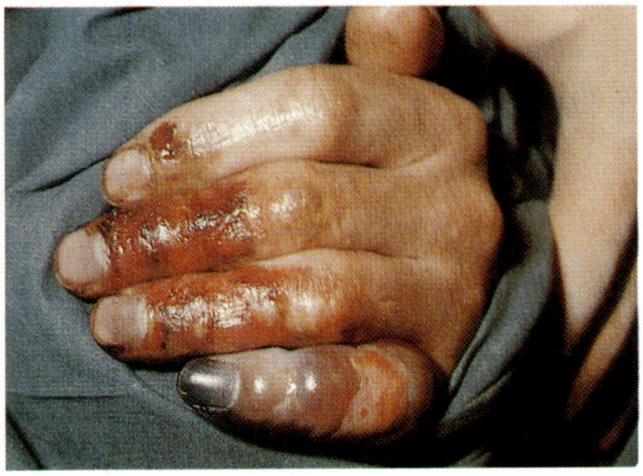

216 Frostbite is seen when there has been freezing of arteries and the tissues by a dry cold, as in this patient, a mountaineer.

217

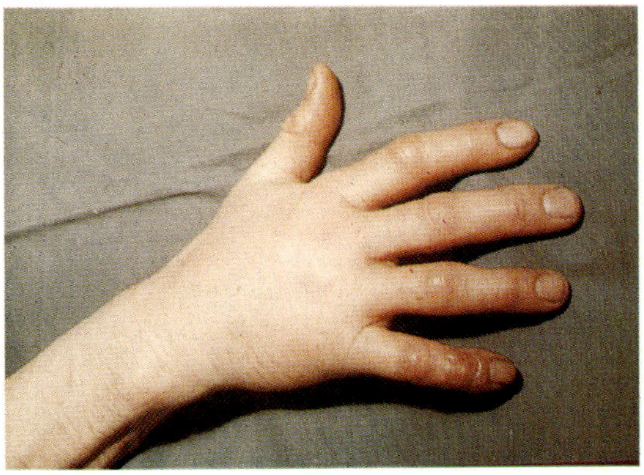

217 Frostbite recovery. A few weeks later with conservative management an excellent recovery was made. In more extreme cases loss of digits is not uncommon.

218

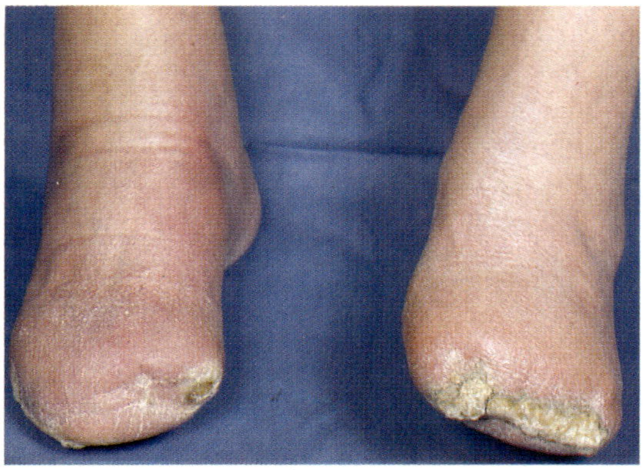

218 In trench foot and immersion foot the exposure is to cold and wet above freezing point. This patient, a soldier in World War I, lost his toes from exposure in the trenches.

7 Arteriovenous fistulae

An arteriovenous fistula is an abnormal connection between an artery and vein. These fistulae may be congenital (multiple or localised) or acquired.

Congenital Arteriovenous fistulae

219

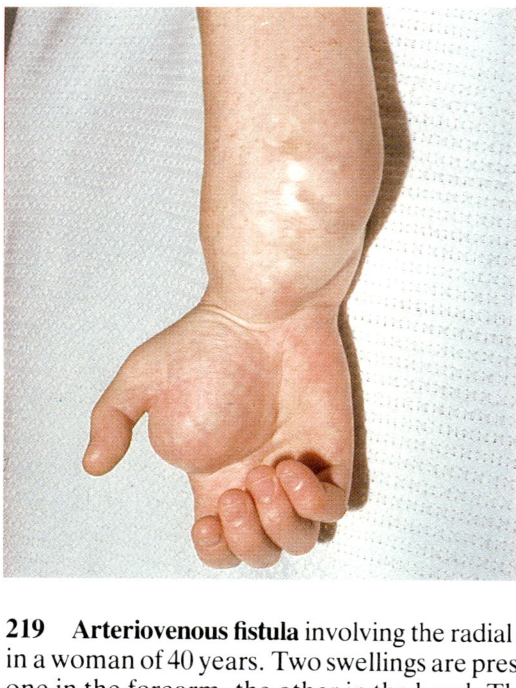

219 Arteriovenous fistula involving the radial artery in a woman of 40 years. Two swellings are present—one in the forearm, the other in the hand. The scar of a previous surgical attempt at closure can be seen. The fistulae here were multiple but no overgrowth of the arm or hand was present. A soft bruit was heard.

220

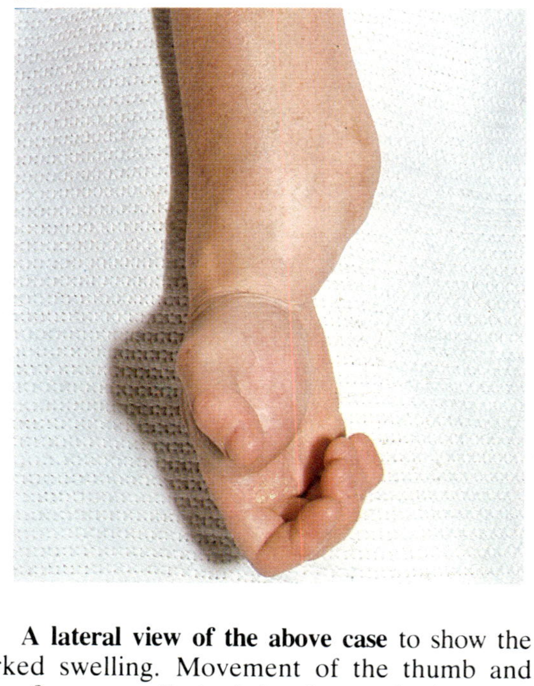

220 A lateral view of the above case to show the marked swelling. Movement of the thumb and index finger was limited, but less so in the other fingers. At a second operation the dilated veins contained much blood clot.

221

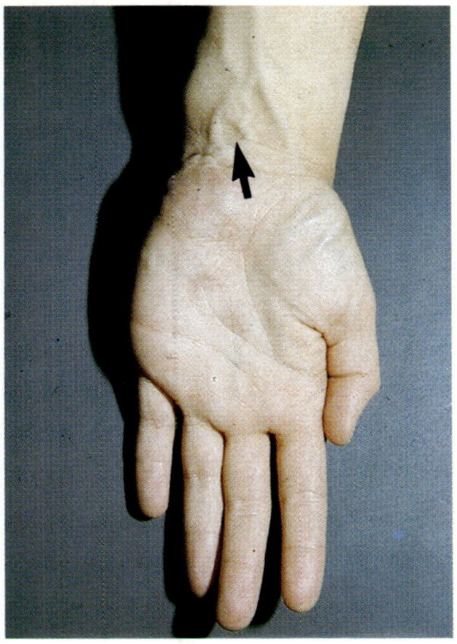

221 Localised arteriovenous fistula. This was a more localised arteriovenous fistula in a teenage girl affecting the hypothenar eminence. The proximal veins are prominent. A thrill was noticeable and a murmur clearly heard. Arteriography was carried out.

222

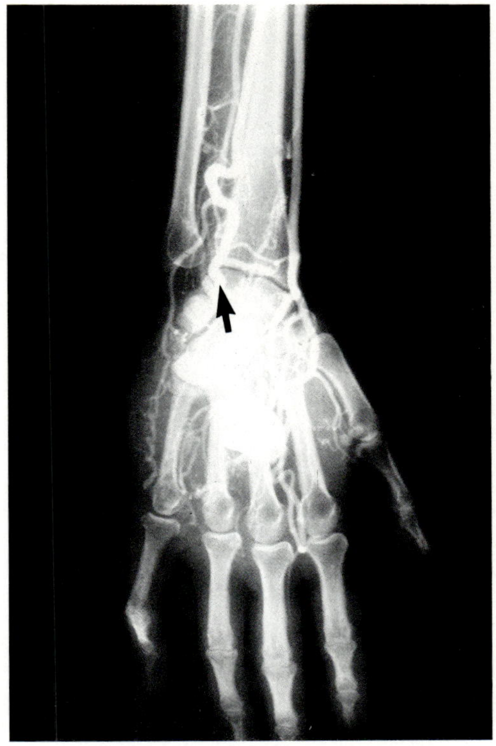

222 Arteriovenous fistula. The angiogram showed a mass of vessels in the hypothenar area. A dilated vein is shown passing up the arm close to the ulnar artery. At operation a fistula was demonstrated between the ulnar artery and vein. Closure of this relieved her complaint.

223

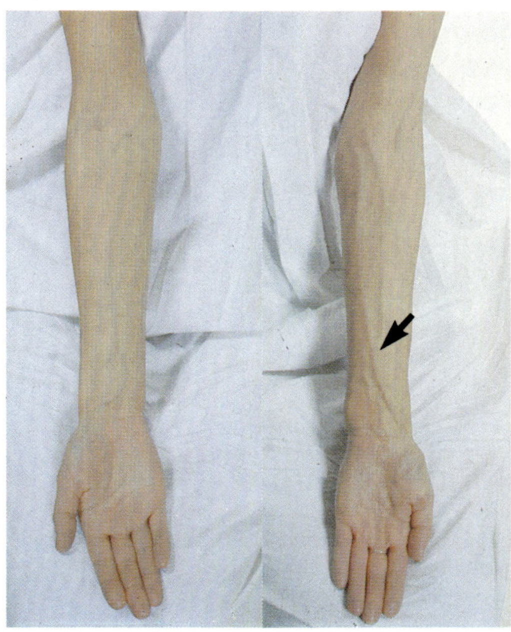

223 Another case of arteriovenous fistula in the left arm shows the marked dilatation of the veins. A thrill was felt and a murmur heard in the veins. These fistulae may lead to lengthening of the affected limb, but not in this case.

224

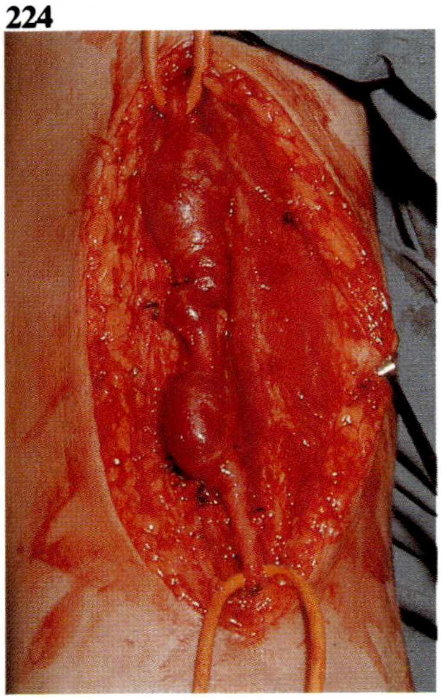

224 Multiple aneurysms. A curious feature of the above case was the presence of multiple aneurysms of the brachial artery. These were saccular and presumably related to a congenital weakness in the muscular wall of the artery.

225

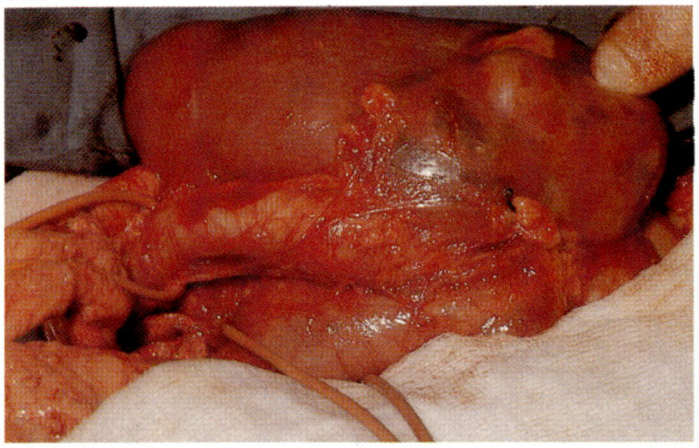

225 Congenital arteriovenous fistula may occur in any part of the body. This patient, a 40-year-old woman, presented with haematuria. Arteriography demonstrated a fistula which was found at operation to be between the renal artery and a very large renal vein, shown with the rubber round it in the lower part of the picture.

226

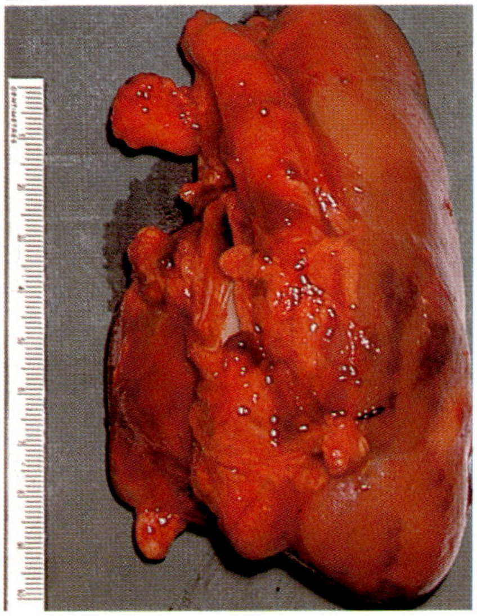

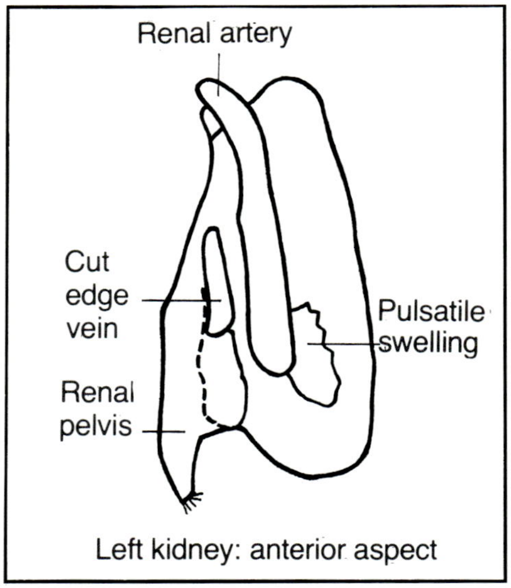

226 Fistula between renal artery and renal vein. The above kidney and fistula is shown with diagram of the fistula.

227

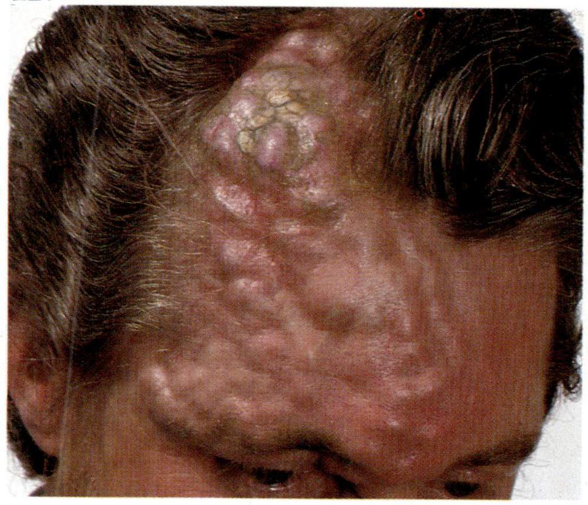

227 Cirsoid aneurysm. This complicated arterio-venous fistula involving the superficial temporal artery and vein with connection with cerebral vessels occurred in this man's teens. It is sometimes termed a cirsoid aneurysm. There was a marked thrill and bruit. Ligation of the right external carotid artery markedly improved the situation, but further surgery with excision of the vessels was necessary.

Acquired arteriovenous fistulae

228

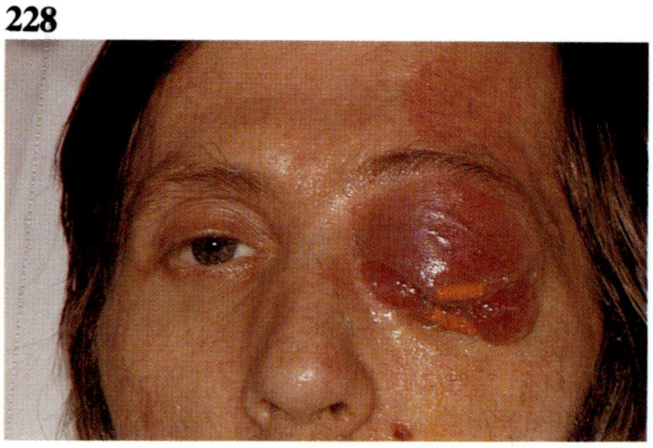

228 Carotid-cavernous fistula may follow a fracture of skull or a rupture of an arterial aneurysm into a vein. The latter was thought to be the case in this man. It produced the classical, if rare, sign of a pulsating exophthalmos.

229

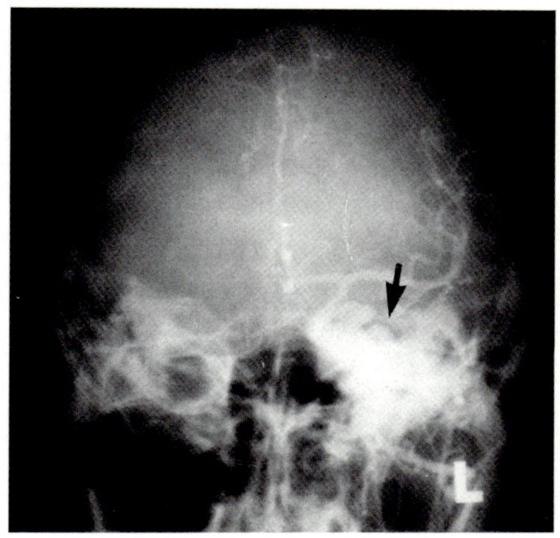

229 Fistula and dilated vessels. An angiogram showed the area of the fistula and the dilated vessels draining it.

230

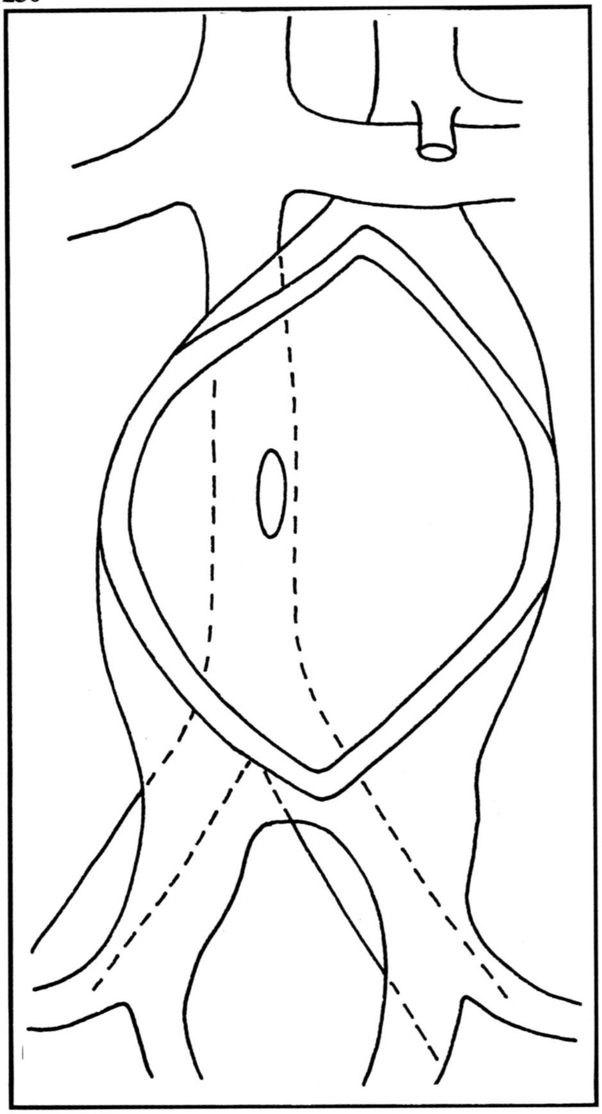

230 Ruptured aortic aneurysm. Rarely an abdominal aortic aneurysm may rupture into the inferior vena cava. The drawing represents the findings at an emergency operation for resection of a ruptured aortic aneurysm. A marked thrill was palpable in the inferior vena cava at operation.

231

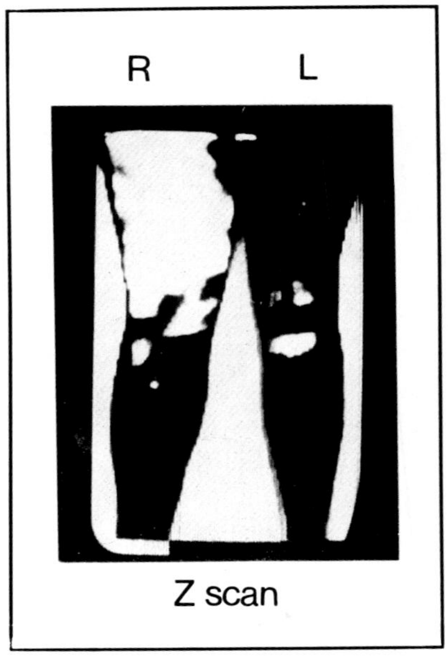

231 Traumatic arteriovenous fistula. Thermography may illustrate the area of increased vascularity in association with an arteriovenous fistula. The white area in the right thigh is the site of a traumatic arteriovenous fistula which followed a knife wound.

8 Tumour of blood vessels

Haemangioma: a) Capillary — port-wine stain
— strawberry mark

b) Cavernous

232

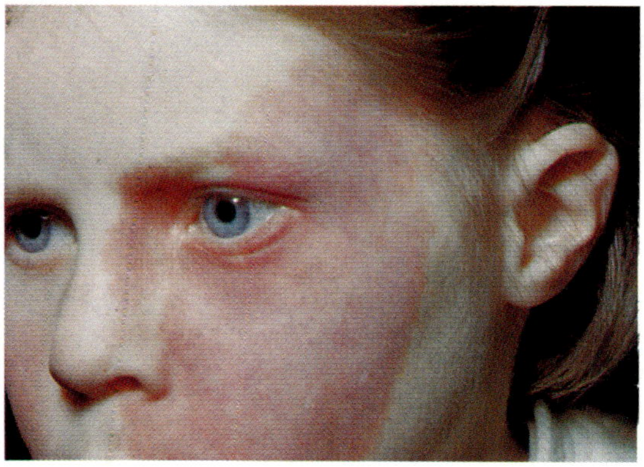

232 Capillary haemangioma. The port-wine stain is a flat slow growing capillary haemangioma. It does not regress but requires excision and skin graft if any treatment is necessary.

233

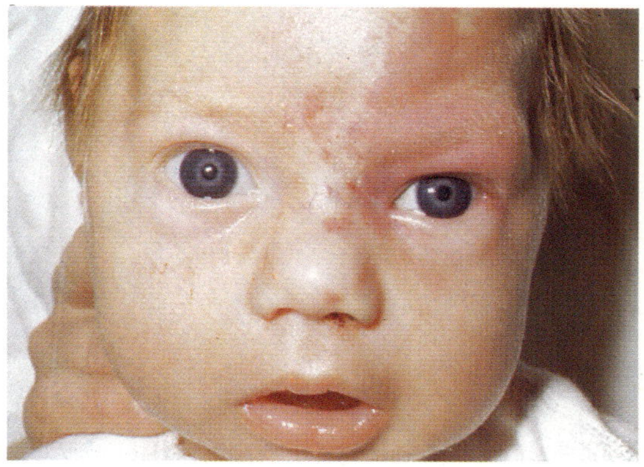

233 Haemangiomata may be associated with similar lesions in neural tissue. In this case the Sturge—Weber syndrome comprises a port-wine stain plus a capillary haemangioma in the meninges and the choroid coat of the eye.

234

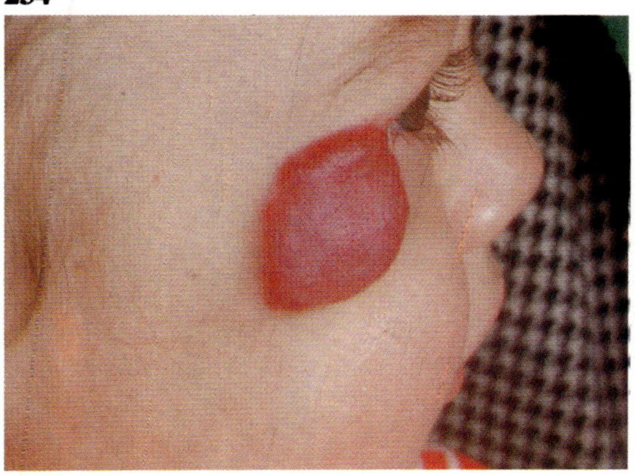

234 The raised or strawberry naevus appears shortly after birth. It grows slowly for months and disappears after a few years. Therefore no treatment is required.

235

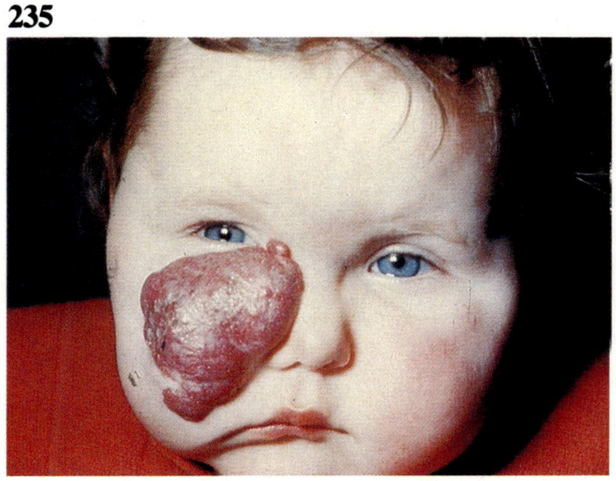

235 The cavernous haemangioma is a soft easily compressible lesion, which may occur in subcutaneous or submucous areas as well as in the viscera. They are composed of large irregular blood spaces.

236

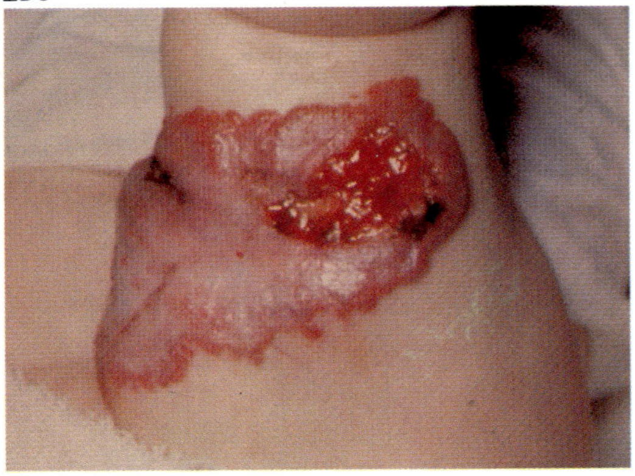

236 A cavernous haemangioma may ulcerate and bleed or become infected. These complications can be serious.

237

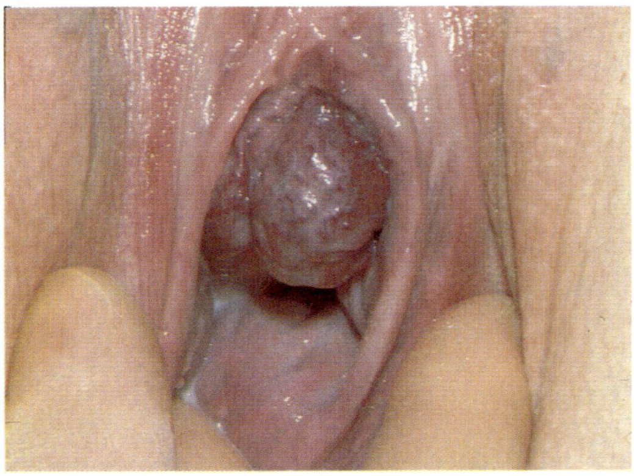

237 This cavernous haemangioma was noted in the vagina in a pregnant woman. It became larger with pregnancy and because it was feared that labour might be dangerous, the haemangioma was removed.

238

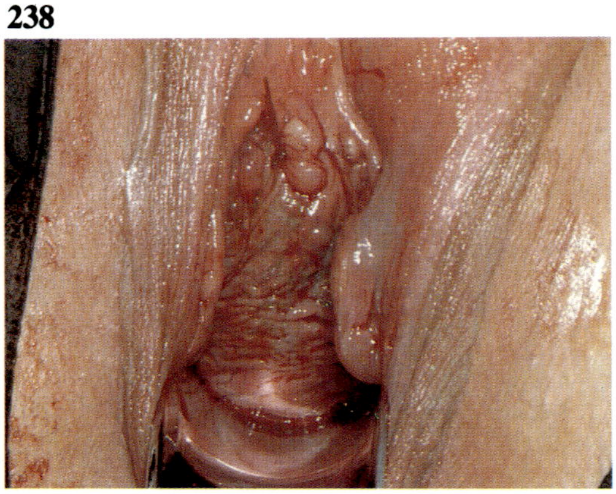

238 The haemangioma was easily excised and labour progressed without problems.

239

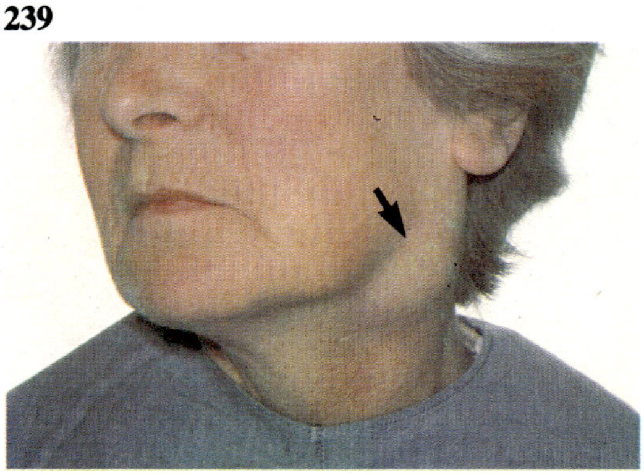

239 A carotid body tumour appears as a symptomless, often long-standing, swelling at the angle of the jaw where it may be mistaken for a parotid tumour or enlarged lymph gland. It is mobile from side to side but not vertically.

240

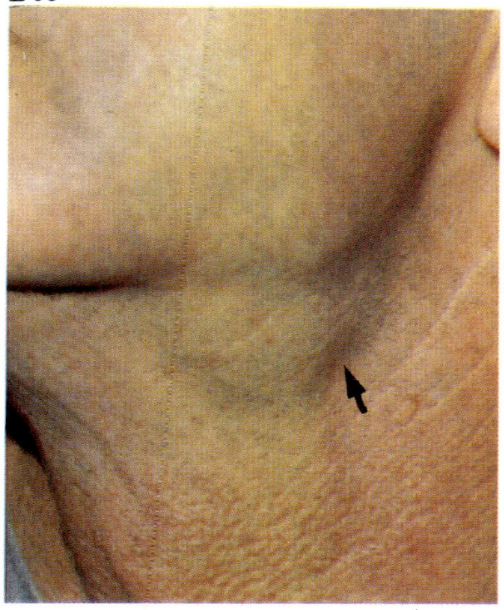

240 Carotid tumour. In this patient the carotid tumour was much smaller than the above and a little anterior to the angle of the jaw. The level was similar—at the bifurcation of the carotid artery.

241

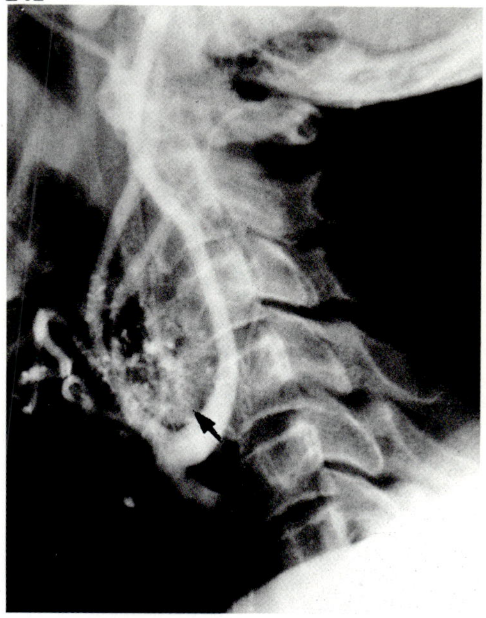

241 Chemodectoma. A carotid body tumour is really a chemodectoma and not a tumour of blood vessels, but they are vascular and very clearly associated with the carotid arteries. Angiogram shows the separation of the carotid vessels by the tumour (goblet displacement) and the blush of vessels in the tumour.

242

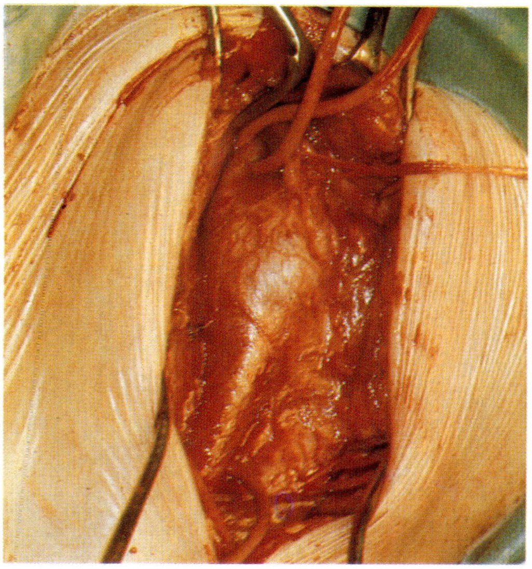

242 A carotid body tumour exposed at operation. The internal carotid artery has a rubber string round it. The tumour arose from the undersurface of the carotid bifurcation to which it was closely adherent. Growth occurs upwards. Transmitted pulsation and a bruit were present but not expansile pulsation. The hypoglossal nerve was close to the upper end of the tumour.

243

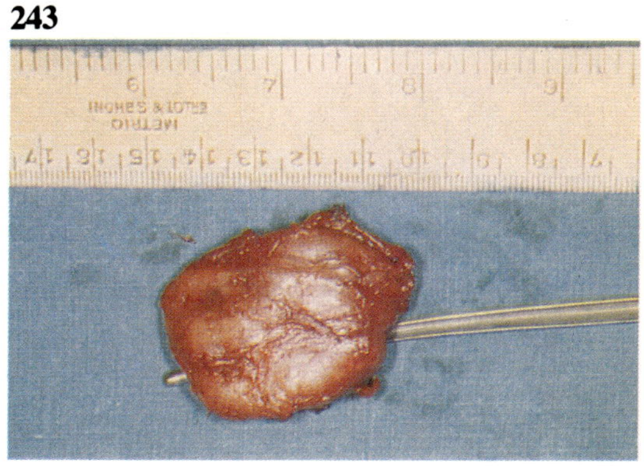

243 An excised carotid body tumour which was well encapsulated. The probe was passed through the external carotid artery which was so involved that its resection made the operation easier.

244

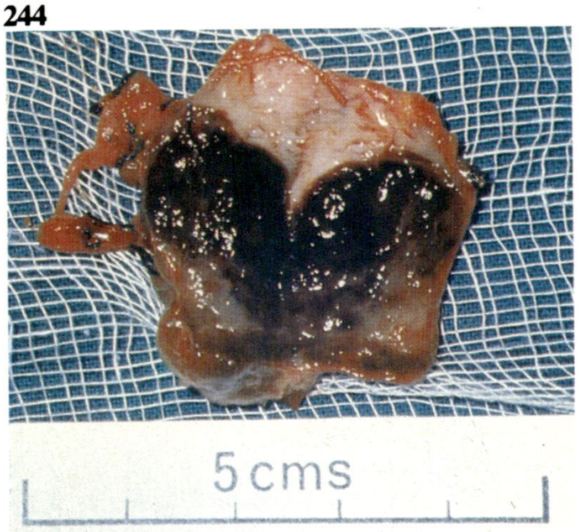

244 Incised tumour. The cut surface of the tumour gives an idea of its vascularity. The tumour may have histological evidence of malignancy but the growth is usually very slow so that resection is not always mandatory. Local invasion is commoner than distant metastases.

245

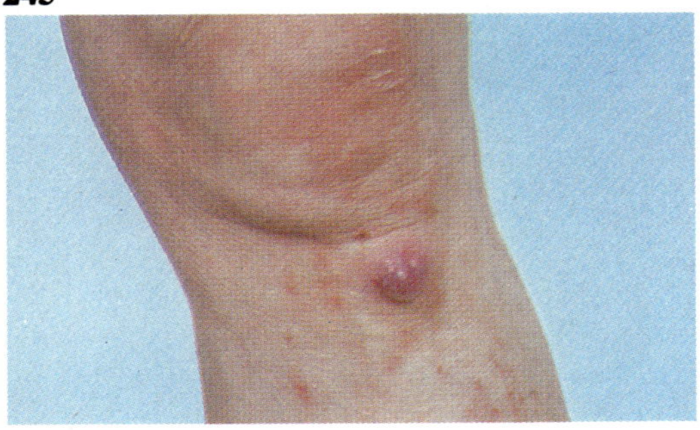

245 A glomangioma (glomus tumour) presents as a painful red/blue swelling in the skin of limb. In this case the swelling below the knee was well localised and curiously tender. Especially in females it may appear under the nails.

246

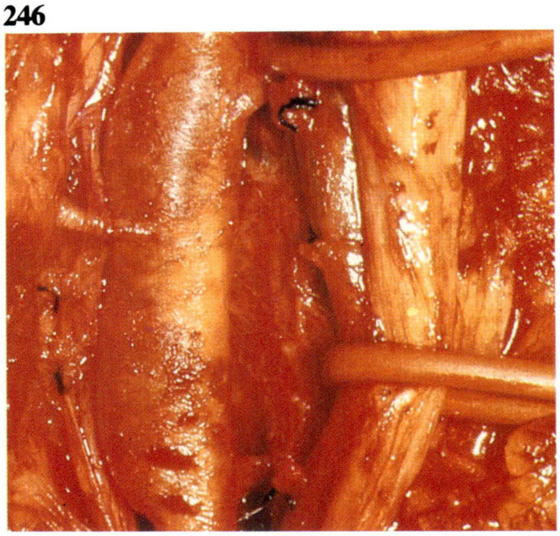

246 Cystic degeneration of the popliteal artery is not really perhaps a tumour of blood vessels. However, the condition is a mucoid cyst of the adventitia in the middle third of the artery. It produces a narrowing of the vessel with claudication. The area is seen at operation as a bulge.

247

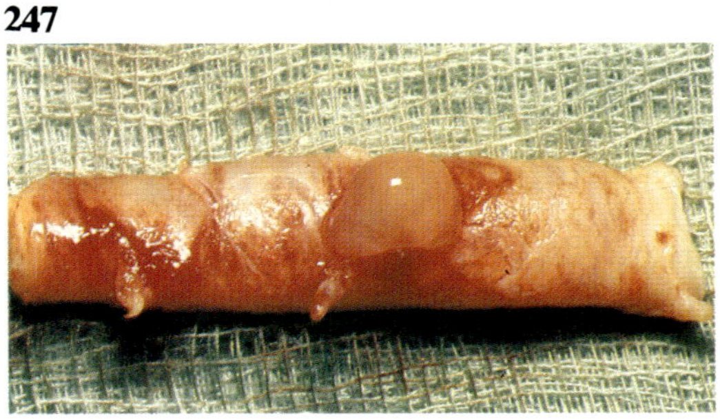

247 Excised cystic area. The cystic area is excised in toto and a graft inserted. The mucoid nature of the lesion is evident.

248

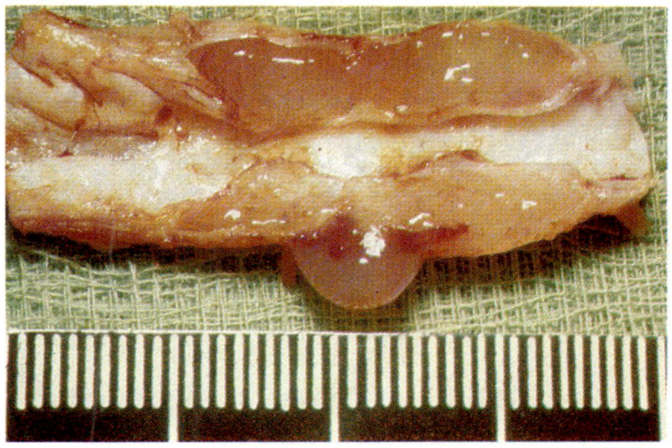

248 Popliteal stenosis. The mucocystic condition is even more evident when the lesion is opened up. The area of popliteal stenosis is evident.

Malignant tumours of blood vessels

These are rather rare and include angiosarcoma and Kaposi's sarcoma.

249

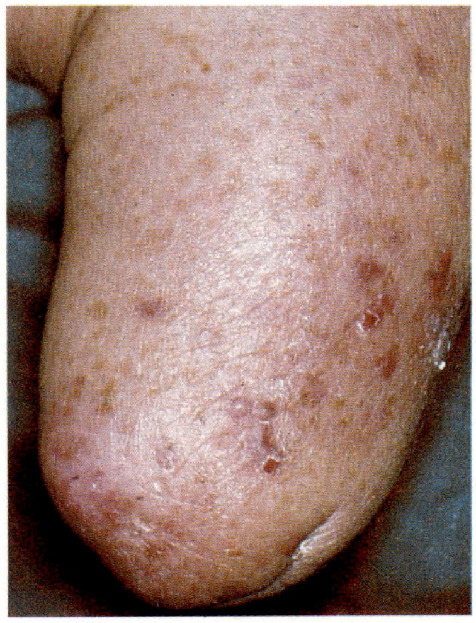

249 A Kaposi's sarcoma is more commonly seen in equatorial Africa than in Europe. It appears as nodular lesions of purple or brown colour. In this case the lesions appeared on an amputation stump. Biopsy establishes the diagnosis.

9 Vascular injuries

250

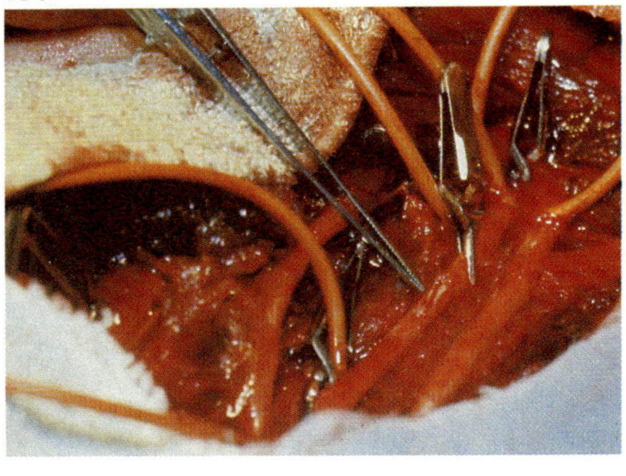

Open injuries

250 Axillary artery injury. Direct injury to the left axillary artery was the result of a stab wound. The hole in the artery is indicated by the forceps. Repair necessitated excision of the damaged portion plus end-to-end anastomosis. The wide exposure enables proximal and distal control.

251

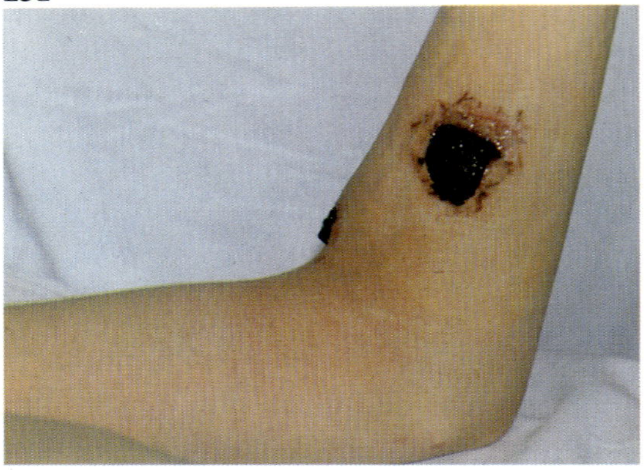

251 Blood clot. This patient had his forearm pierced by a wedge of glass. The entry wound is full of blood clot. Exploration of the wound failed to reveal the injury to the artery. Recurrent bleeding ensued with further exploration.

252

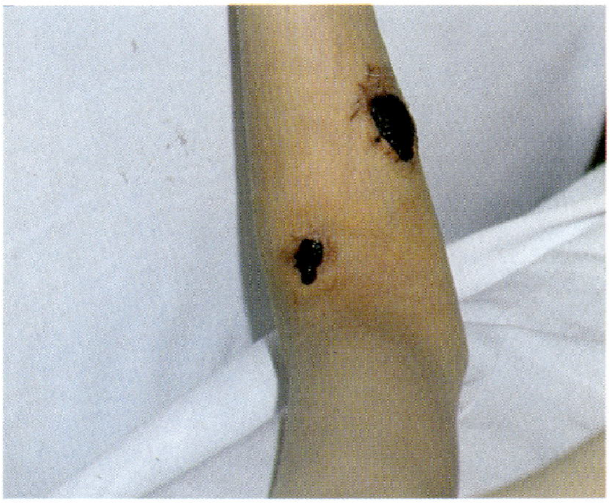

252 Elbow contracture. The entry and exit wounds are visible, both full of clot. Contracture of the elbow is beginning to take place. The clot was visibly pulsating—pulsating haematoma typical of a false aneurysm.

253

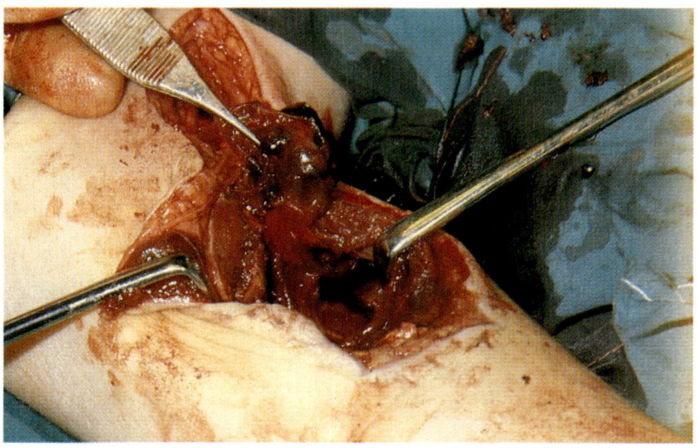

253 False traumatic aneurysm. Exploration revealed the false traumatic aneurysm indicated by the forceps. This rose from a branch of the artery to the muscle. The cavity which contained the aneurysm is under the retractor on the right. Haemorrhage had been contained by the fascia.

254

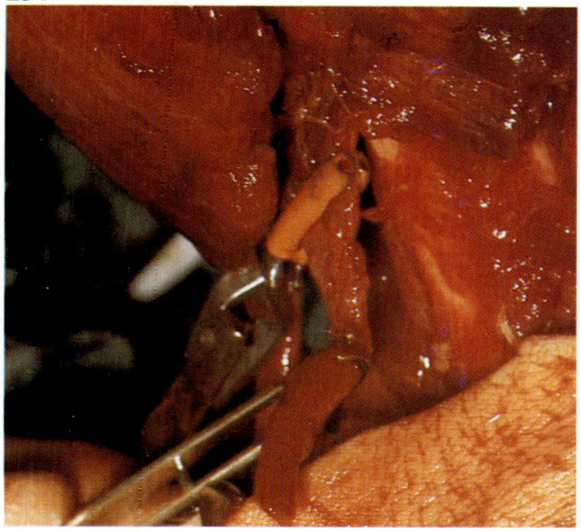

254 Complete transection of the brachial artery is illustrated. The artery had sealed itself off by contraction and thrombosis. The artery is held up by the forceps.

255

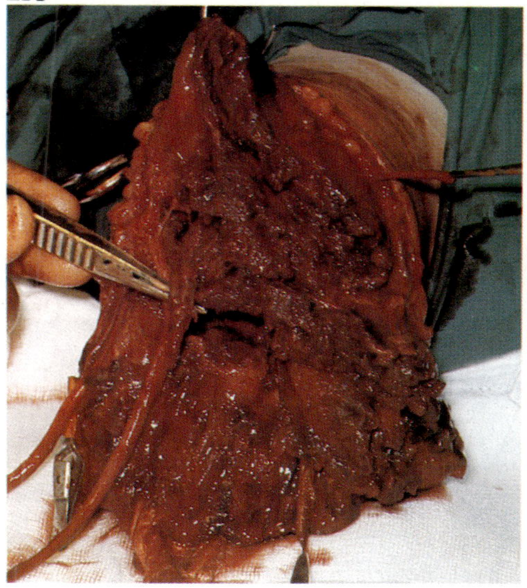

255 Traumatic amputation of the arm illustrates the grossest form of arterial injury. All vessels were torn across. The artery had sealed spontaneously. The artery is on the dissecting forceps.

256

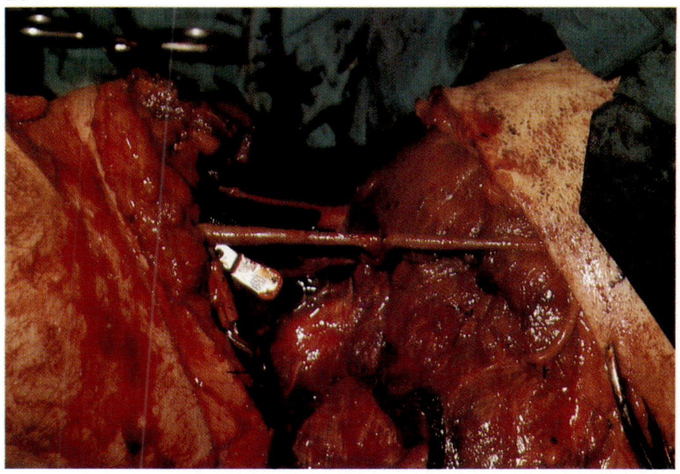

256 Re-implantation of arm. This figure shows one of the steps in re-implantation of the amputated arm. The bones were fixed first, then the veins shown here were anastomosed and finally the arteries.

257

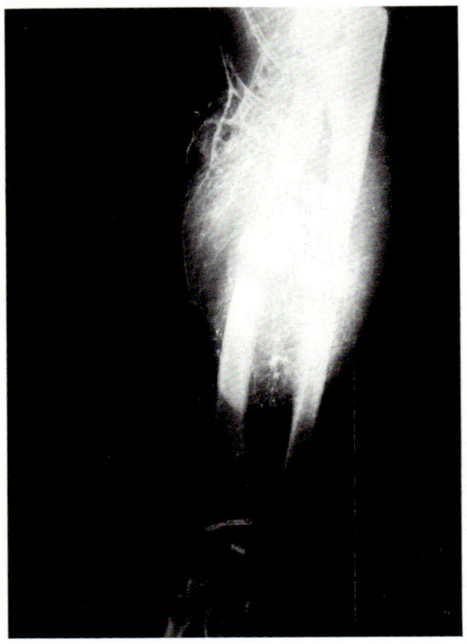

257 A crushing injury was sustained on the forearm. No pulses were felt at the wrist. Arteriogram shows a massive bleeding in the forearm with spidery vessels at the wrist. This is virtually a compression injury possibly with some vasospasm but also much disruption of the vessels.

258

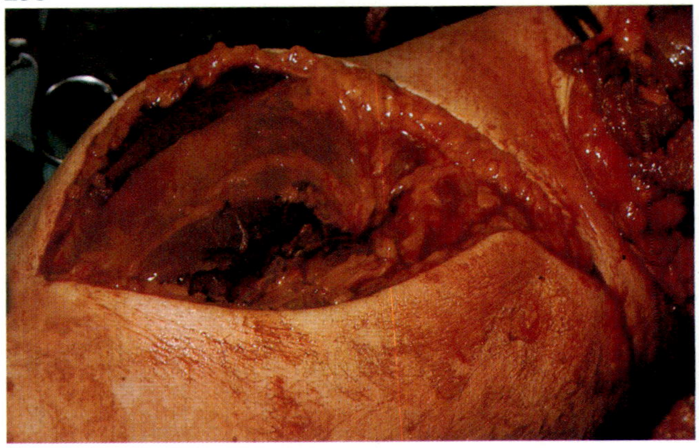

258 Incision of the forearm revealed the very tight fascia enclosing clot under pressure. The even less severe case, if untreated, would lead to ischaemic contracture.

259

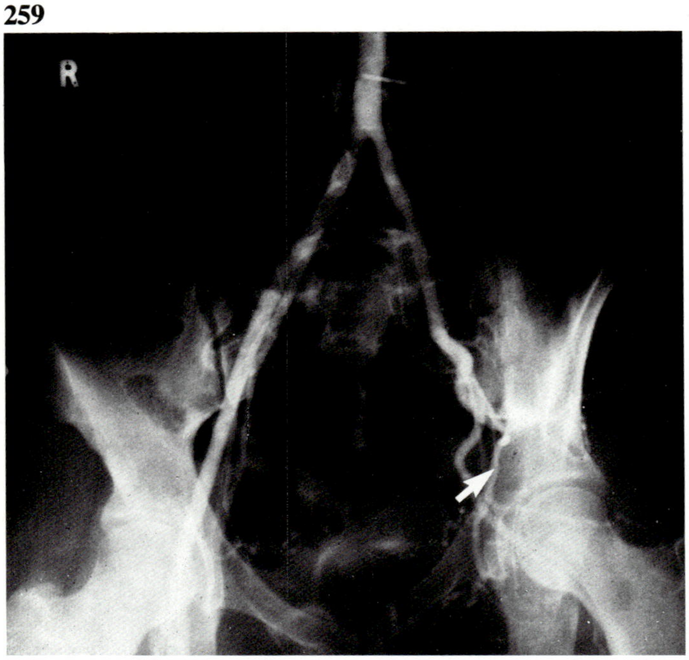

259 Thrombosis. This patient had her left femoral artery cannulated for open heart surgery. The hole was sutured but damage to intima and narrowing had produced thrombosis with, on arteriogram, a block in the vessel. A subsequent graft was required.

260

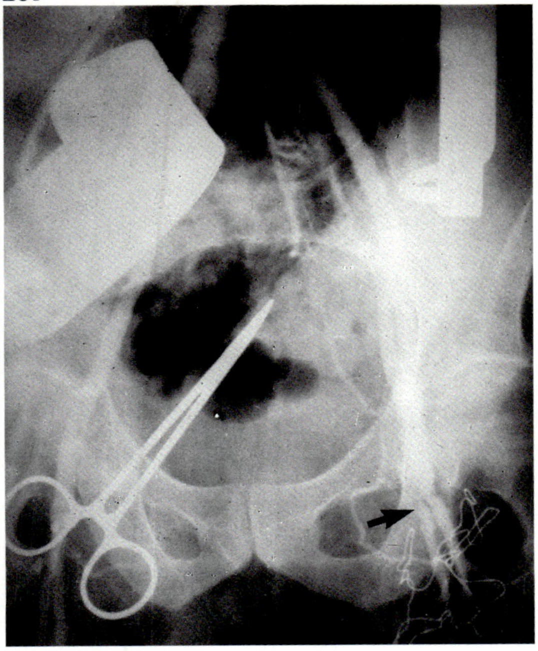

260 Intimal tear with curling up of the intima is shown. An aortofemoral graft had been inserted into the left common femoral artery. Lower pulsation was not good and operative arteriogram showed the narrowed area at the top end of the superficial femoral artery just above the radio-opaque thread in a gauze swab. The artery was reopened and the intima tacked down.

261

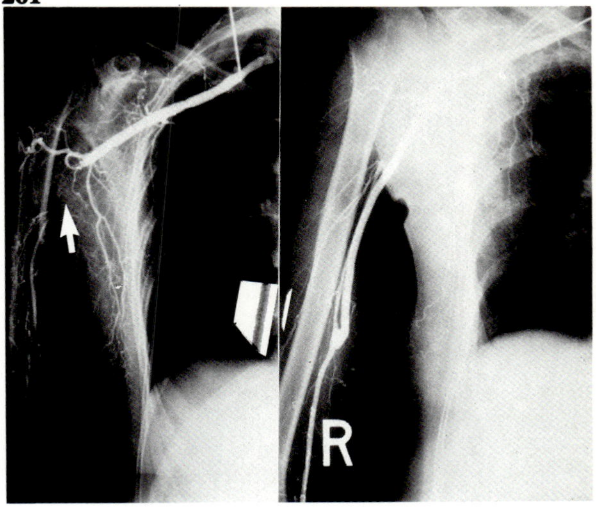

261 Post-mastectomy radiation. A rare form of damage caused by radiation after mastectomy for cancer of the breast, ten years previously. A gradual onset of forearm claudication occurred a few months before the arteriogram, which shows a block in the axillary artery in the left figure and its correction by vein bypass on the right.

262

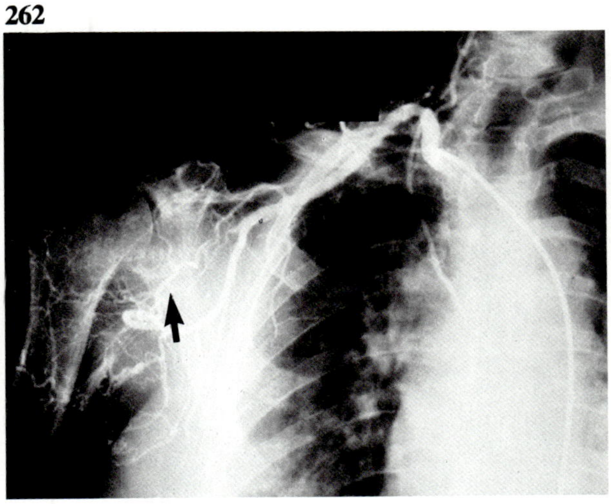

262 Artery catheterisation damage. Intimal damage can also result from brachial artery catheterisation in arteriography. This produced a block in the artery itself due to thrombosis. This route is less commonly used now.

263

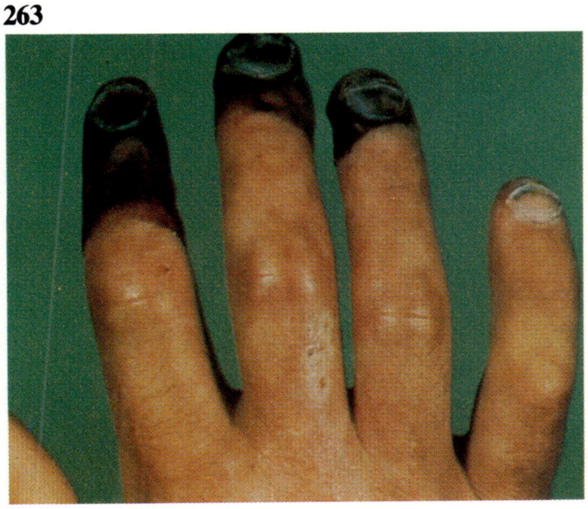

263 Chemical irritation of intima. Intra-arterial injections may produce a chemical irritation of the intima with thrombosis. This man was a drug addict who unfortunately put the injection of drugs into the artery at the elbow.

264

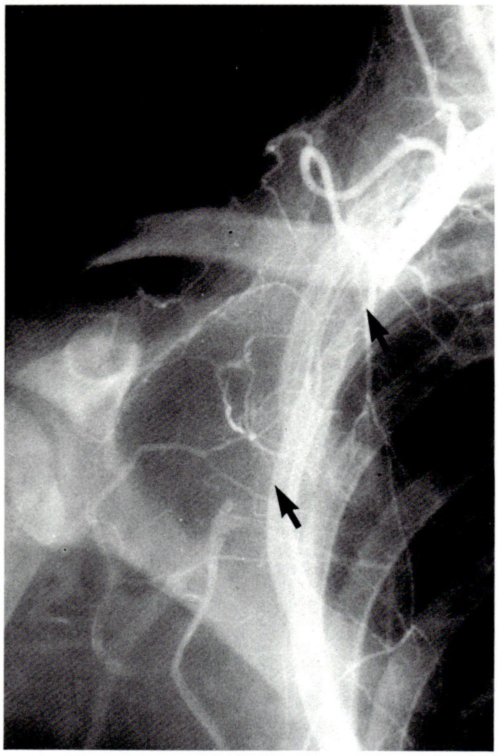

265

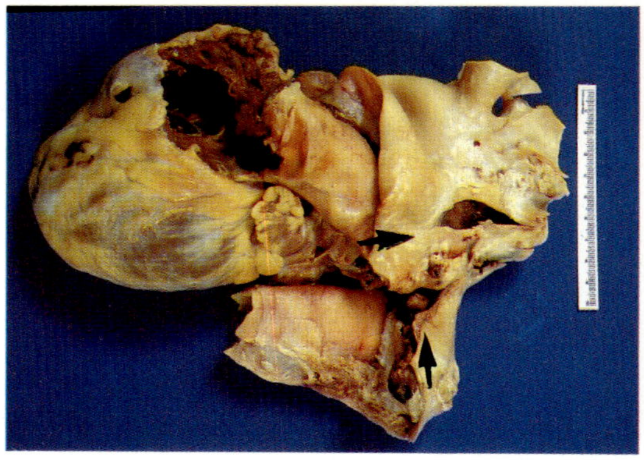

265 Tear in the aorta arch may occur in association with road traffic accidents. The illustration shows a gross injury with rupture of right ventricle, tear of the arch and aorta beyond the subclavian artery as indicated by arrows. Death was instantaneous in this case. In lesser cases there may be increasing broadening of the mediastinal shadow on xray and possibly a bloody effusion in the left chest.

264 Hyperextension injury may cause intimal tear and thrombosis without external arterial rupture. This boy had a motor cycle accident with brachial plexus avulsion injury and axillary artery thrombosis. The skin circulation remained good and exploration was not required.

266

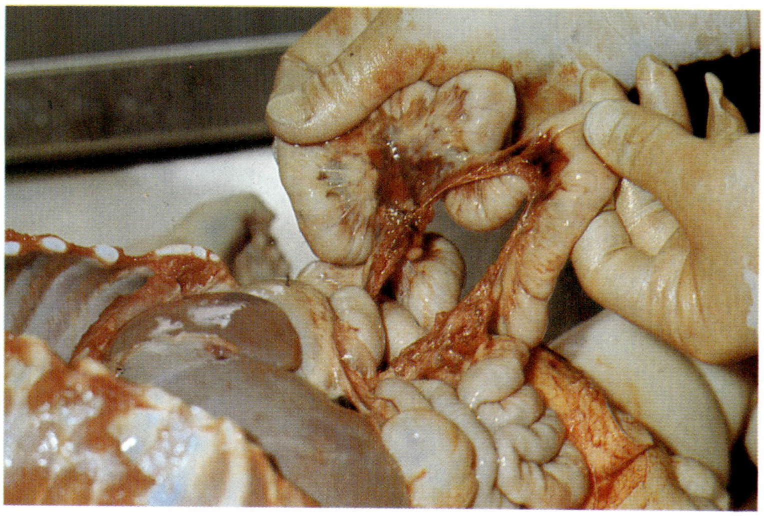

266 Ruptured mesentery. Closed injury to vessels can occur from blunt abdominal trauma, which in this case has ruptured the mesentery of the small intestine and torn the vessels. The child died.

10 Veins

Venous disorders may be classified into:

1 Congenital abnormalities of veins
2 Varicose veins
3 Deep vein thrombosis

Congenital abnormalities

Congenital abnormalities are rare. They are broadly of two types: angiomata of veins (phlebangioma) or dilated venous trunks (phlebectasia). More common is the arteriovenous fistula, which must be excluded by the absence of a thrill and murmur in the veins and arteriographic evidence of a connection.

267

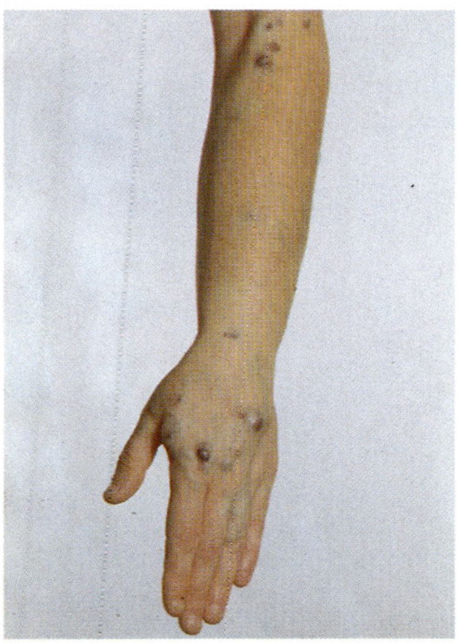

268

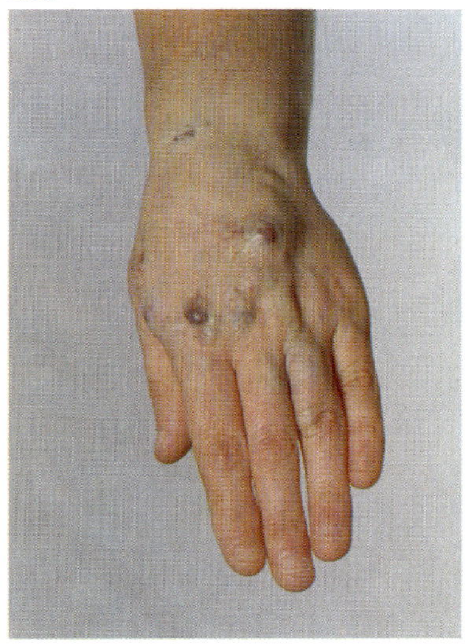

267 Phlebectasia in the arm of a 40-year-old woman. She had noticed prominent veins in the left arm since childhood. Overgrowth of the limb was absent. In the dilated veins are prominent areas of thrombosis.

268 The angiomatous areas on the dorsum of the hand are prominent.

269

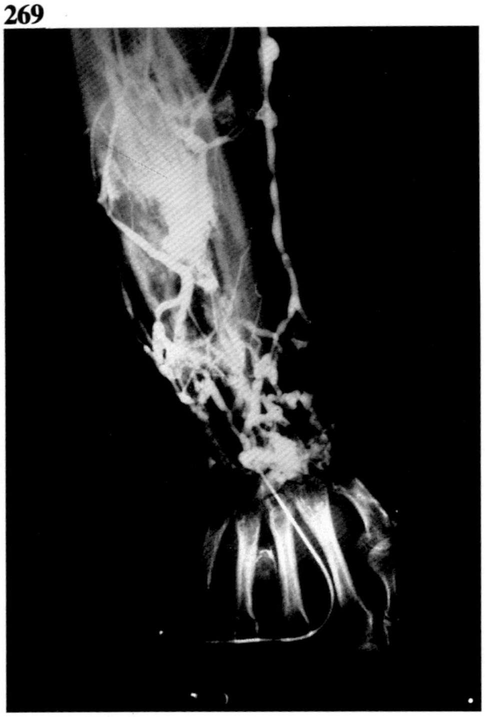

270

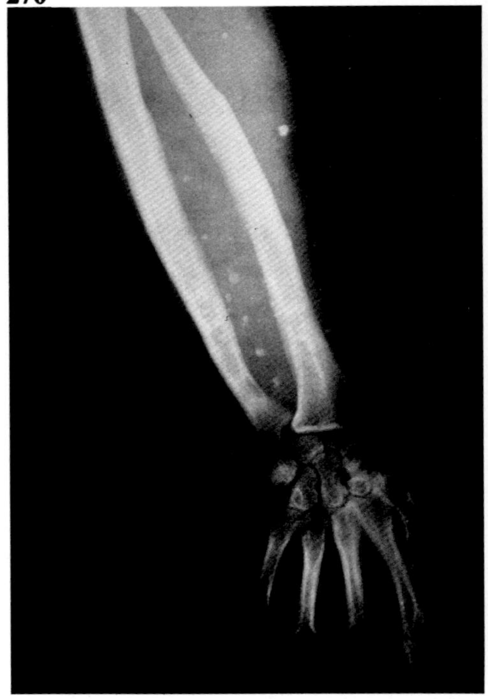

269 Dilated veins. The venogram demonstrates the dilated veins with sàccular areas and the angiomatous collection over the wrist.

270 Calcification. As in long-standing areas of thrombosis calcification has taken place and is visible on plane x-ray.

Varicose veins

Varicose veins are of two types: *primary* varicose veins where the underlying cause is unknown, possibly a congenital defect in the wall of the vein, as a family history is frequently present, and *secondary* varicose veins where there is backflow from deep to superficial veins from incompetent valves in the connecting veins or in the upper end of the long saphenous vein. Valves may be damaged by back pressure from increased pressure in deep veins as in pregnancy or by direct trauma, external injury, infection (thrombophlebitis), or as a result of deep vein thrombosis.

271

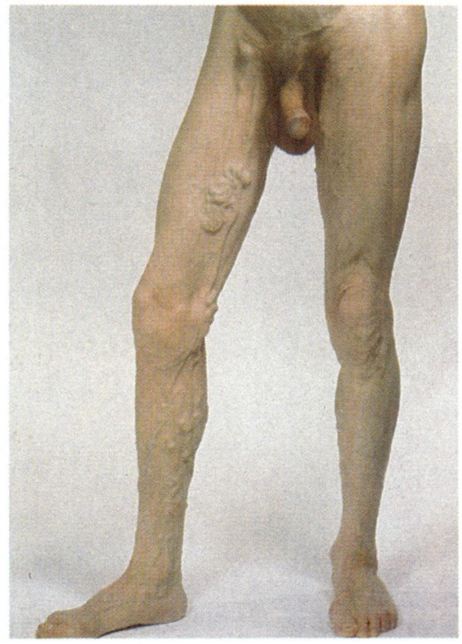

271 Primary varicose veins with tubular like dilatation of the long saphenous system and areas of tortuosity in mid-thigh, behind the knee, and upper calf, where one should suspect and look for possible incompetent perforators.

272

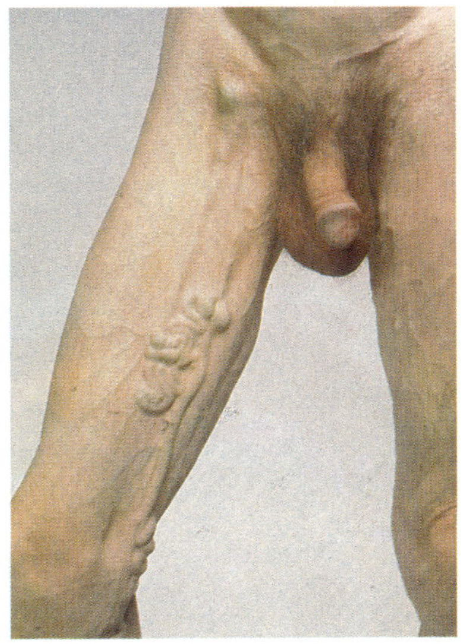

272 A varicocele. A close-up view of above showing the marked dilatation of the saphenous vein at its upper end—a varicocele. There was a strong family history of varicose veins.

273

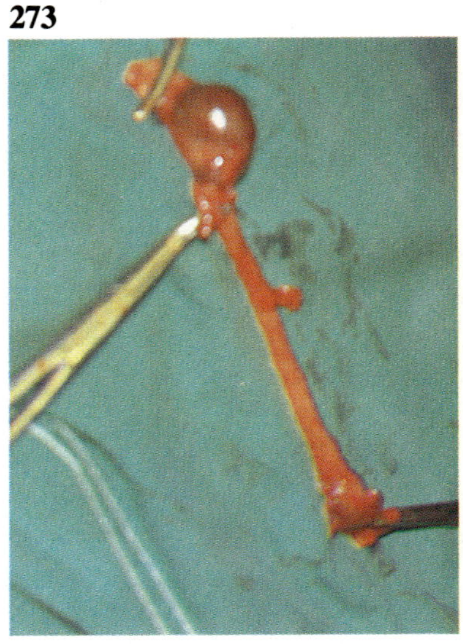

273 Excised saphenous vein. The upper end of the long saphenous vein was excised. The variocele is clearly seen as in a further dilatation at the lower end.

274

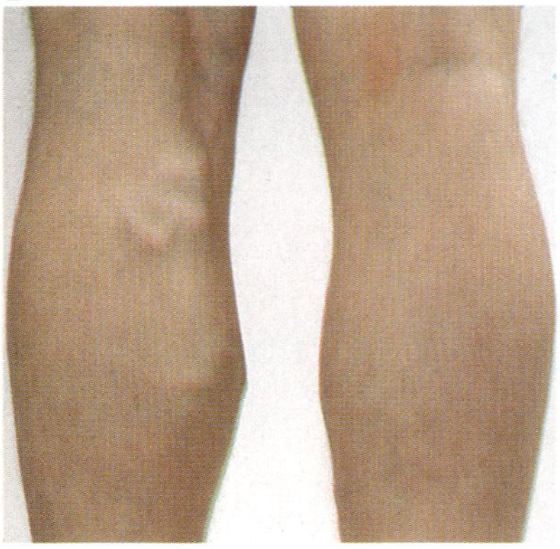

274 Short saphenous system. The short saphenous system is rarely involved in the varicose state. Most veins even on the posterior aspect of the legs fill from the long saphenous system. In this case the varices were cured by ligation of the short saphenous system.

275

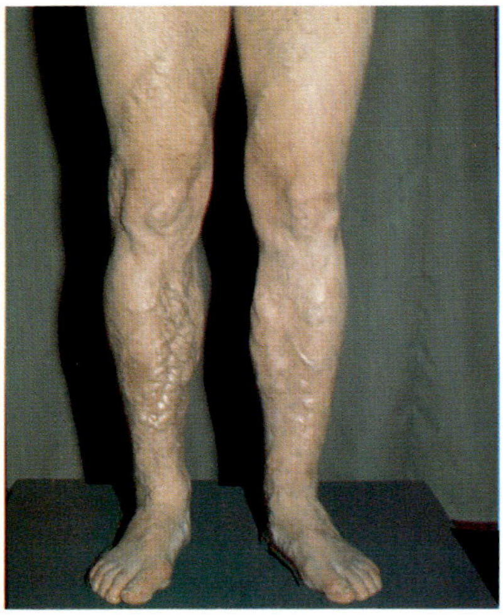

275 Varicose veins may be very extensive in both legs. Note extensive thigh vein involvement in the right leg.

276

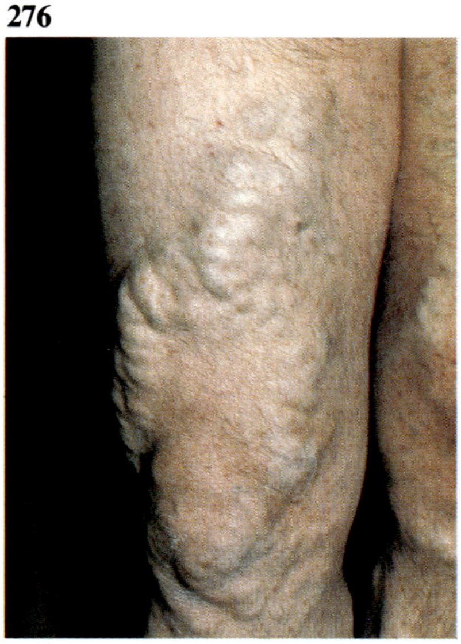

276 Dilated and tortuous veins. The thigh veins not normally noticeable can, in varicose conditions, become enormously dilated and tortuous and spread down both sides of the knee. They seem to be especially susceptible to thrombophlebitis.

277

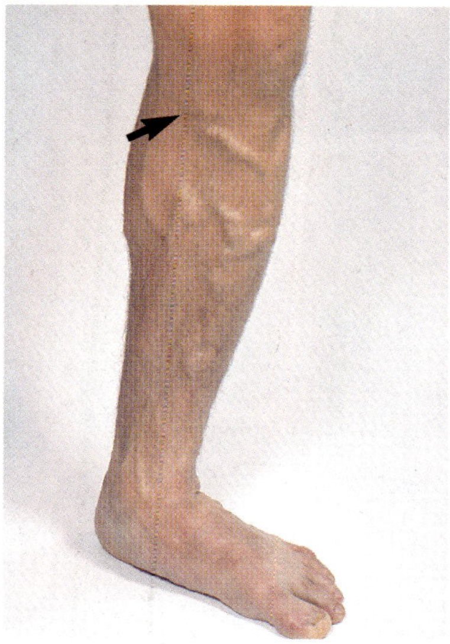

277 Varicose veins may be prominent below the knee with no evidence of trouble higher up. The leaking perforator was found, at operation, behind the slight bulge visible at the proximal end of the vein.

278

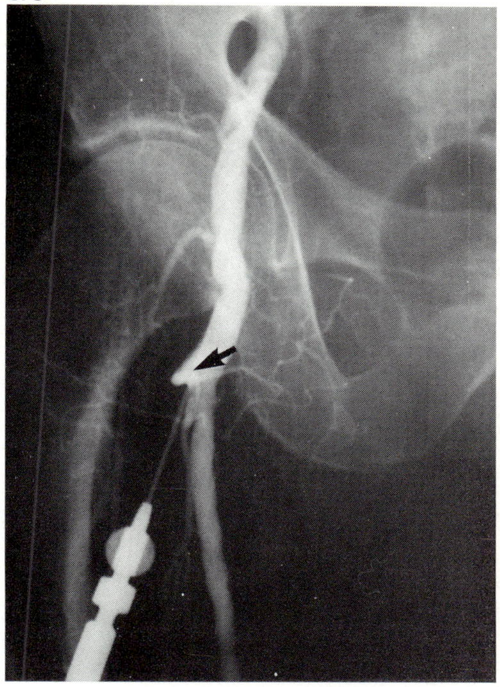

278 Valve competency. A normal venogram with the proximal end of the long saphenous vein as it enters the common femoral vein just lateral to the needle. This illustrates the competency of the valve at the upper end of the long saphenous vein.

279

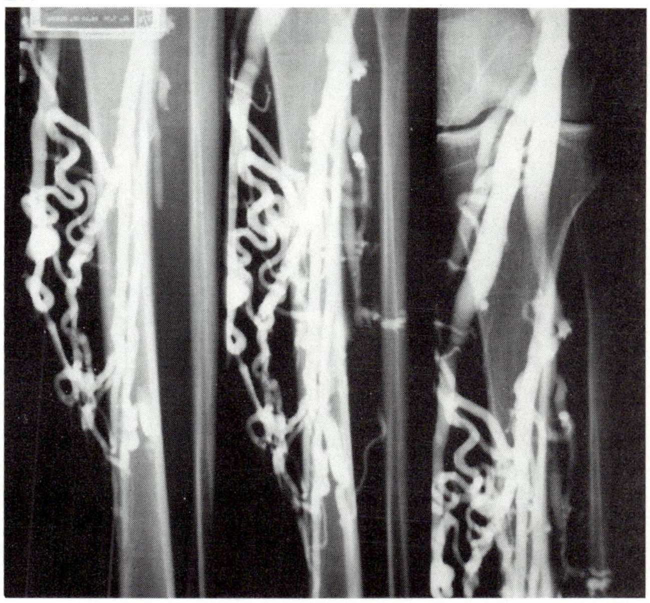

279 Incompetent veins. Below the knee the incompetent veins are seen joining the deep to superficial veins.

280

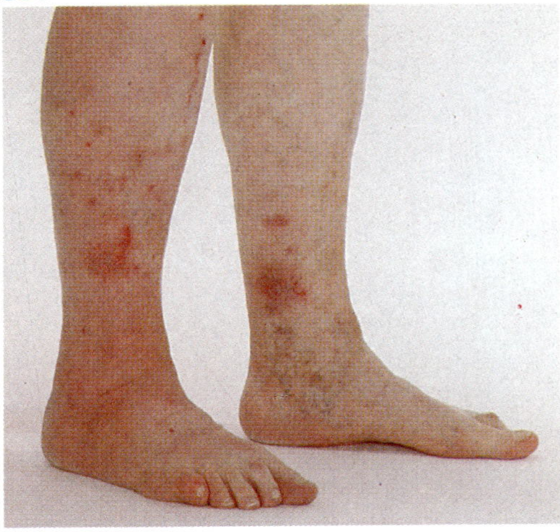

280 Cellulitis of the lower leg is a particular complication of long-standing varicose veins. The areas are red, painful and tender. Both legs were affected—the right worse than the left.

281

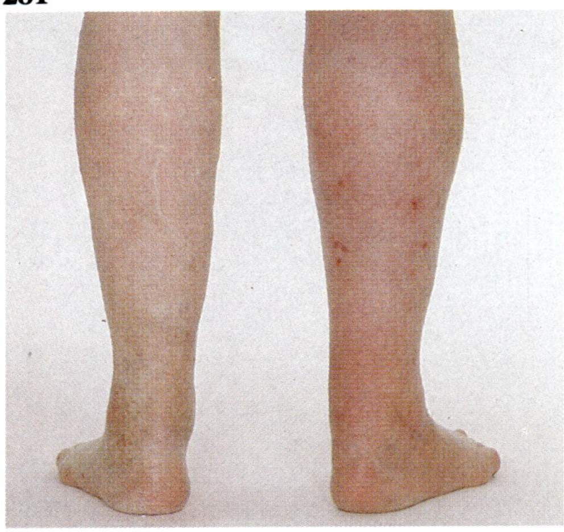

281 Cellulitis. The posterior view showed up the heightened colour in the right leg where there is greater thickening of the ankle. Cellulitis of this type does not quickly respond to antibiotics and often recurs.

282

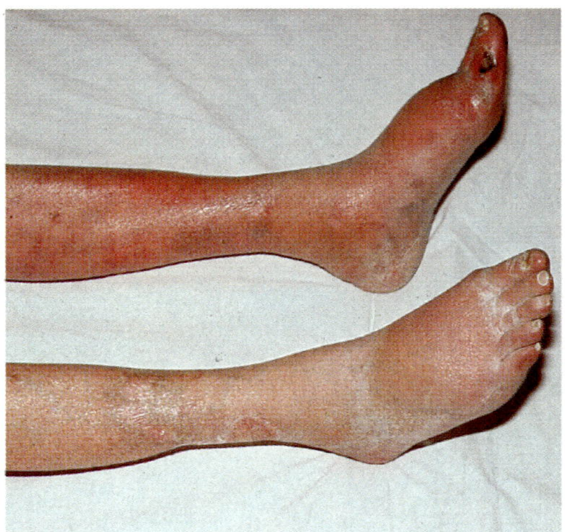

282 Varicose ulceration. This 70-year-old lady had a long history of varicose veins with ulceration of both legs. The left one in particular was affected by cellulitis. The gross oedema of both feet was partly due to the venous problems but it also reflects the dependency oedema associated with severe rest pain from associated occlusive arterial disease.

283

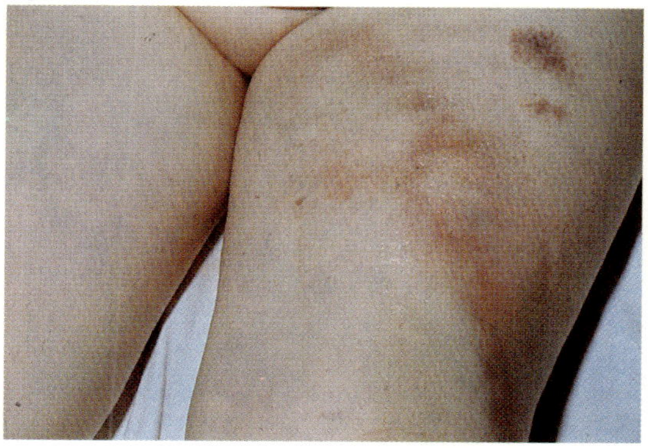

283 Superficial phlebitis is also a common complication of varicose veins shown here in the anterior thigh veins—a common site. Migration of clot to the lungs is not common with phlebitis but it can occur. Inflammation affecting valves will render them incompetent, so increasing the incidence of varicose veins.

284

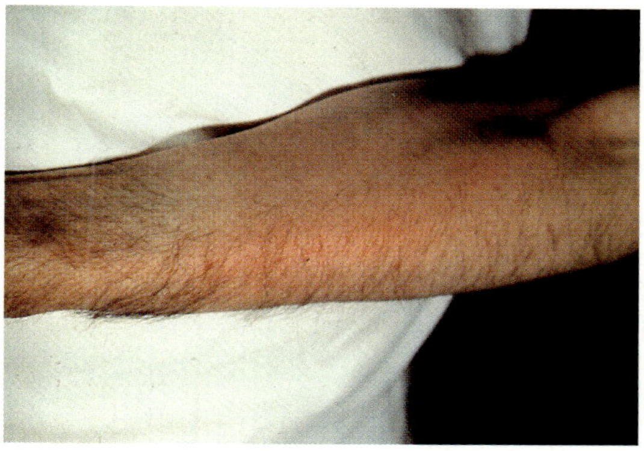

284 Phlebitis can, of course, occur without varicose veins as in this patient who had an intravenous infusion put up in the arm vein.

285

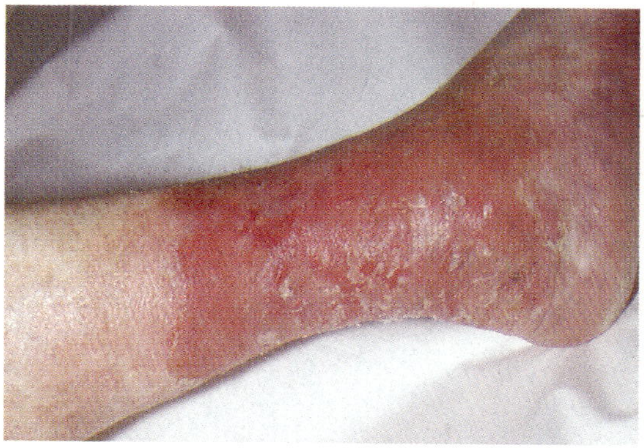

285 A varicose dermatitis may be present especially in the inner side of the lower leg. The relatively acute looking condition is possibly an allergic response to the various ointments and lotions used in the dressing.

286

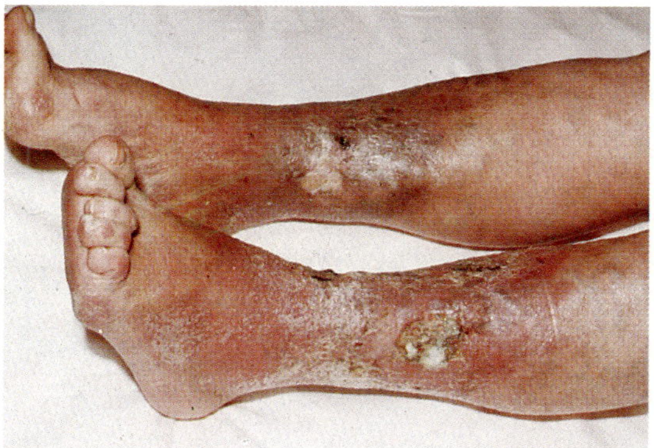

286 Long-standing varicose dermatitis has a brownish colour and may be seen with a varicose ulcer in the common site in the lower leg. Incompetent perforators may be demonstrated by venography just above the ulcer or in the floor of the ulcer.

287

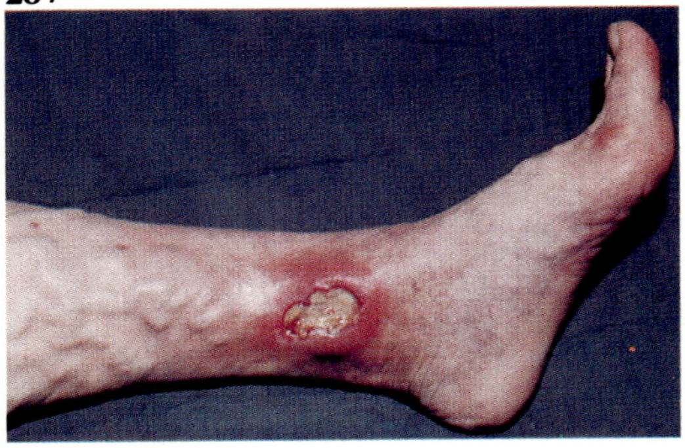

287 A typical varicose ulcer is demonstrated with the obvious varicose veins. These are not always so prominent. The ulcer will respond to simple measures plus elimination of the veins.

288

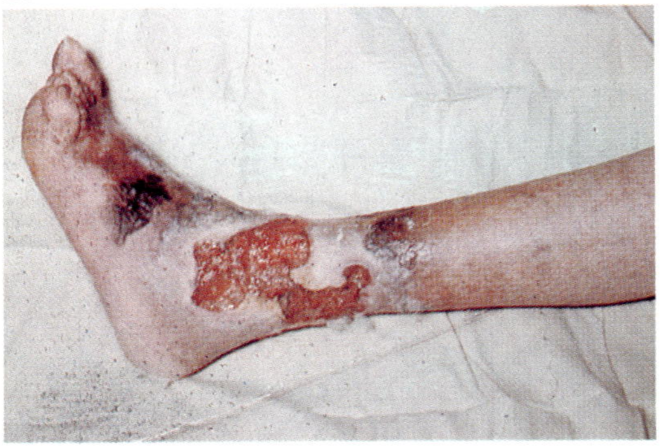

288 Varicose ulcers. The ulcers can however, become extensive, infected and difficult to clean up. Skin grafting may be required.

289

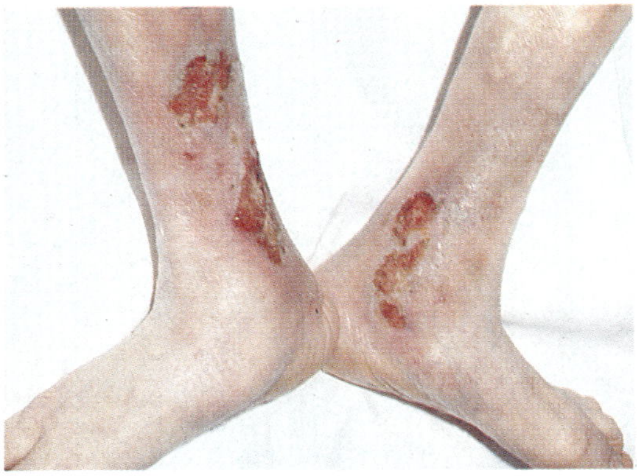

289 Bilateral ulceration is common as are bilateral veins. These ulcers are gradually healing with pressure dressings. Incompetent perforators should be sought.

290

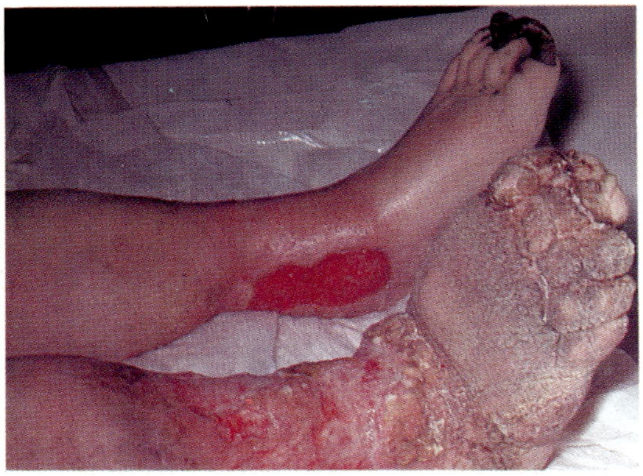

290 Gravitational ulcers are secondary to deep vein thrombosis and are particularly resistant to simple measures. They may heal only to breakdown again. This is an extreme example affecting both legs with an 'elephant's foot' appearance in the right foot due to secondary lymphatic stasis as a result of circumferential ulceration.

291

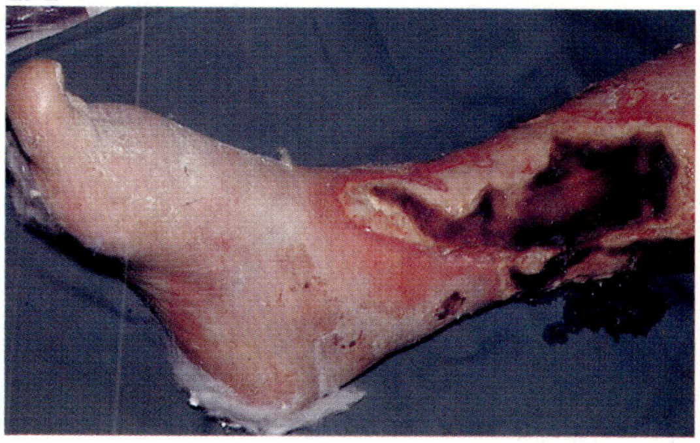

291 Ulceration in the medial side of the leg may be iatrogenic. This patient had an operation of ligature of perforating veins above the ankle. In the elderly and with too extensive undermining of flaps, the skin can be devitalised.

292

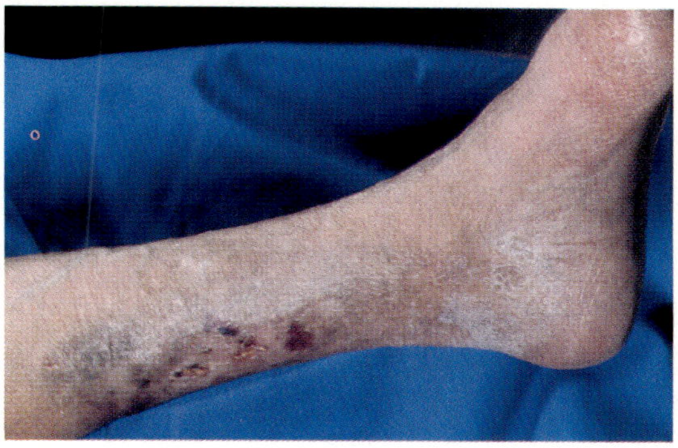

292 Pigmentation and ulceration. This 72-year-old lady had varicose veins for many years. The brownish pigmentation was widespread. The veins felt very hard and where ulceration had occurred a white chalky material was present.

293

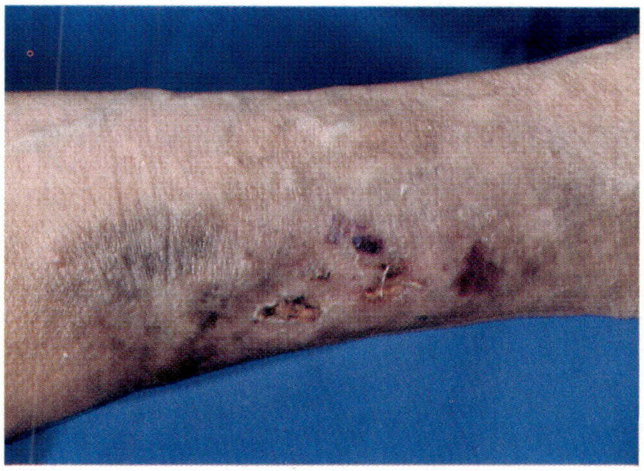

293 Calcification. Closer inspection shows the calcified material in the veins. This most probably resulted from recurrent superficial phlebitis, thrombosis, and calcification of the thrombus.

294

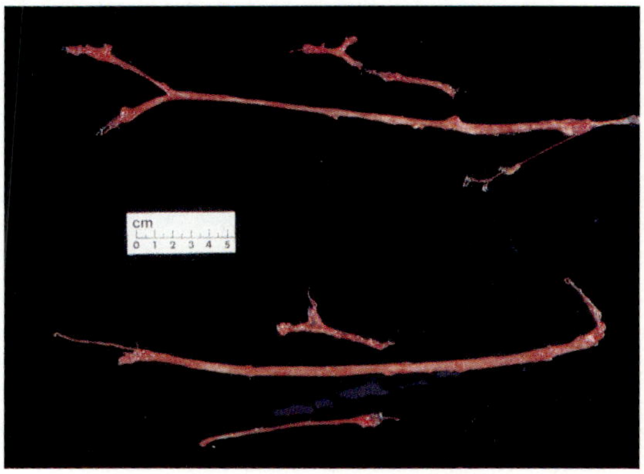

294 Stripping of varicose veins is one of the many methods of treatment. This illustrates bilateral stripping of the veins from groin to ankles and excision of side veins.

295

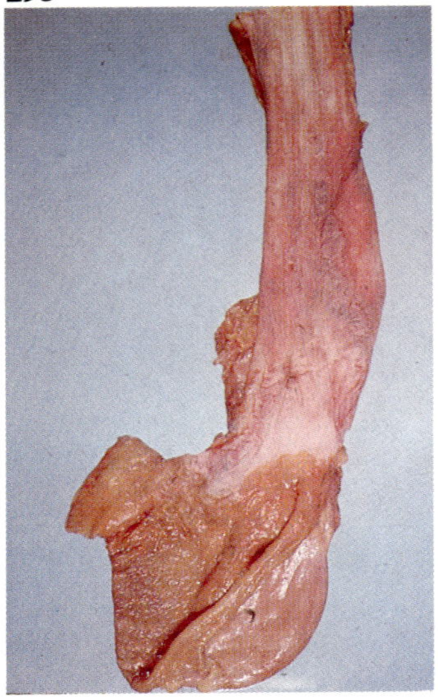

295 Varicose veins can also occur in other areas such as oesophageal varices as shown here, piles and as a varicocoele of the spermatic cord.

Deep vein thrombosis

Deep vein thrombosis may occur with or without presence of varicose veins.

296

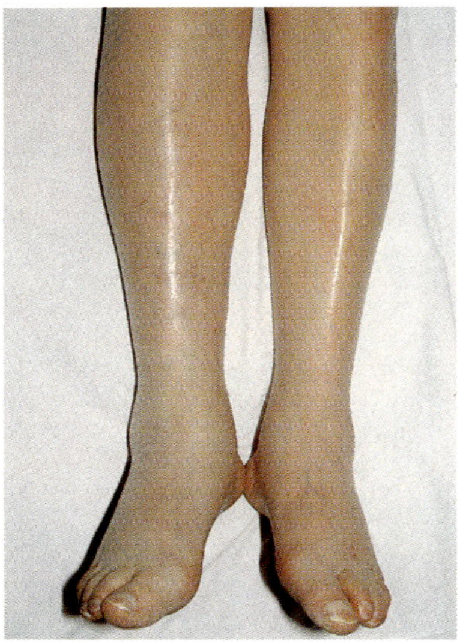

296 Phlegmasia alba dolens. The painful white leg of deep vein thrombosis is illustrated here in the right leg. This developed six days after operation. Pitting oedema was present. The patient responded to elevation of the leg and compression.

297

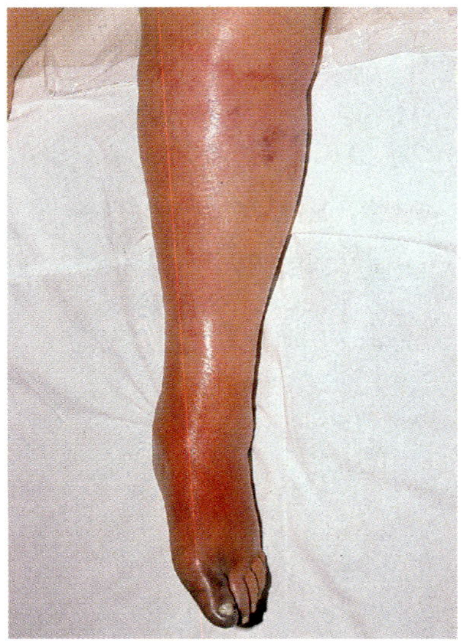

297 Phlegmasia caerulea dolens is the painful blue leg where the whole limb has a reddish-blue colour due to arterial stasis as a result of compression and rarely thrombosis of the artery due to the great tissue pressure. This may go on to gangrene unless the pressure is relieved by thrombectomy.

298

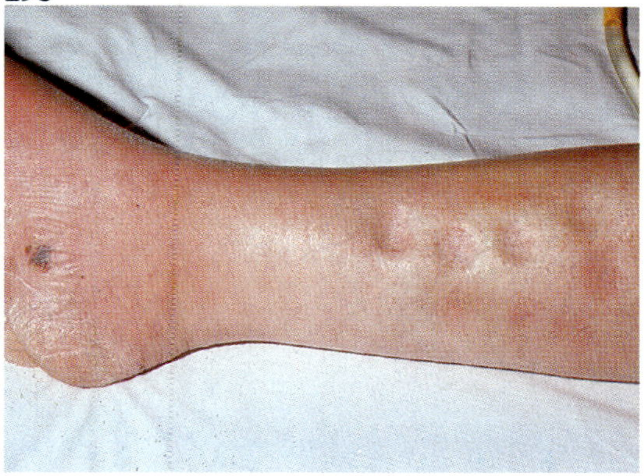

298 Gross pitting oedema is demonstrated in such cases.

299

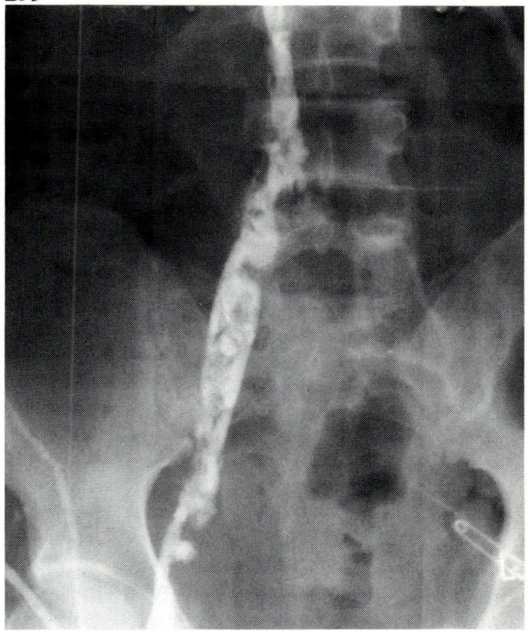

299 Contained thrombus. Venography is the standard technique for demonstrating the site and extent of the venous thrombosis. The iliac veins show the mottled appearance of contained thrombus.

300

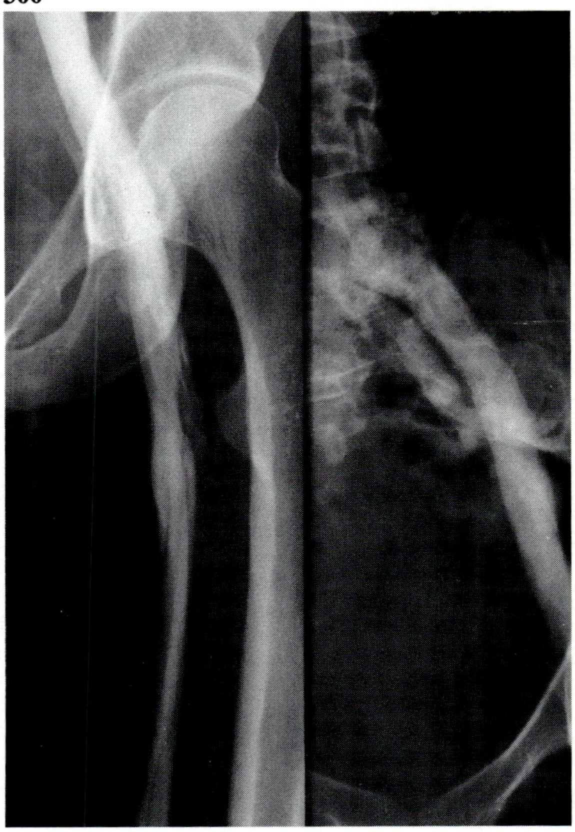

300 Normal venogram. This is contrasted with the smooth appearance of a normal venogram in this area on the other side, which should also be demonstrated by venography at the same time as the condition is frequently bilateral.

301

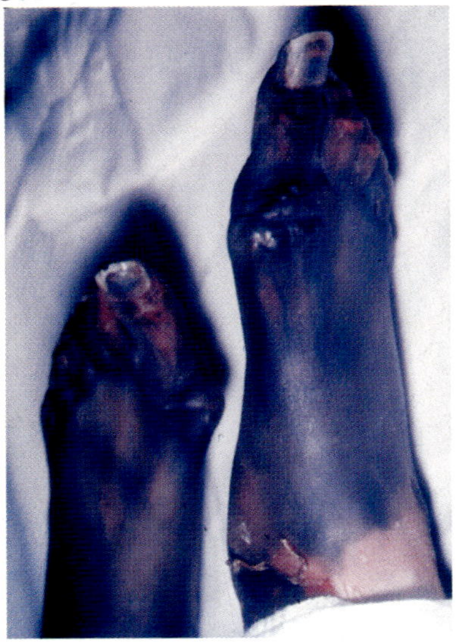

302

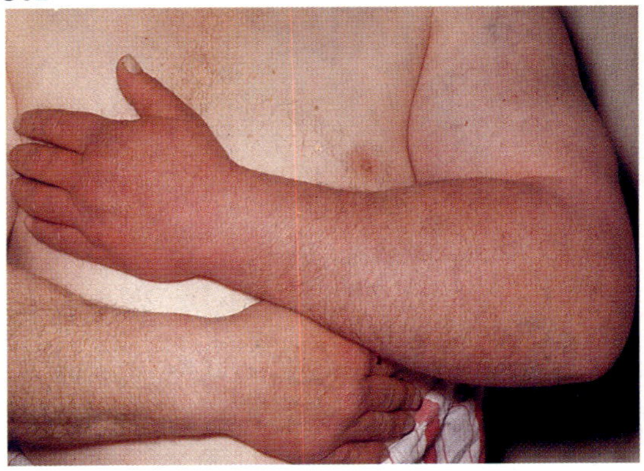

302 Venous thrombosis can also occur in the upper limbs. In this 56-year-old man the swelling came on quickly in the left arm. The arm became bluish-red.

301 Gangrene after venous and arterial blockage. In the most severe form the gangrene after venous and arterial blockage may be bilateral producing a dry and moist form. Toxaemia was most marked in this patient who died before amputation.

303

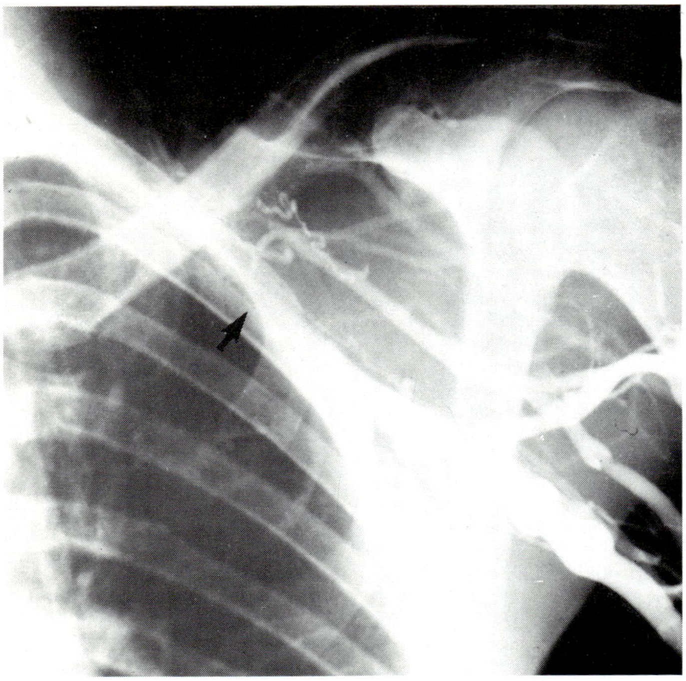

303 Axillary vein blockage. Venography showed extensive blockage of the axillary vein. The cause was unknown. Because he had been working with his arm upright while he painted, it was assumed that cervical outlet compression may have played a part.

304

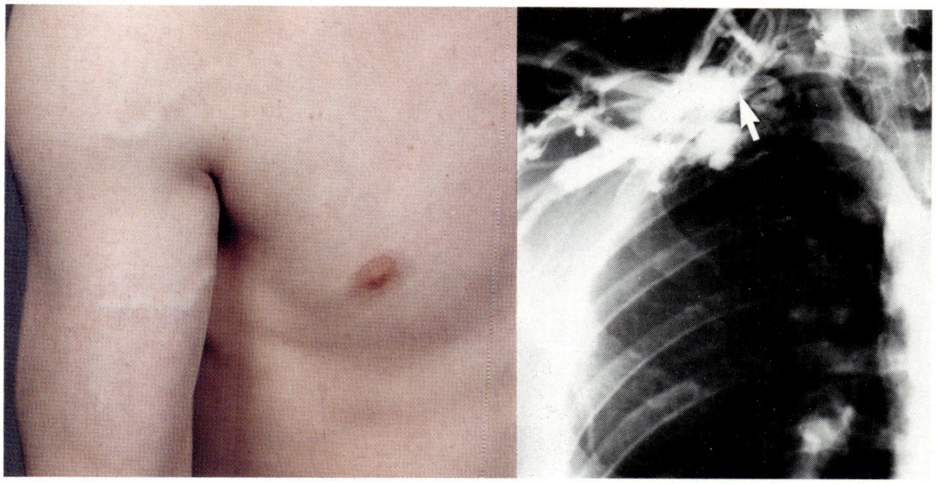

304 Axillary vein blockage. This 24-year-old man had three attacks of swelling of the right arm. On each occasion this swelling gradually disappeared. Venography showed blockage of the axillary vein. Note distended arm veins. Possibly due to cervical outlet compression—the 'effort syndrome'.

305

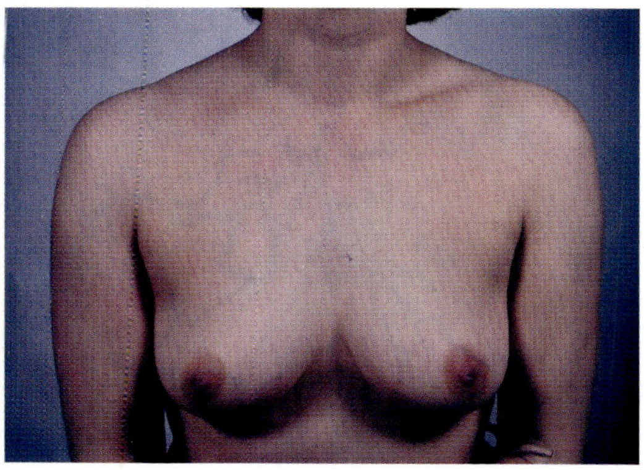

305 Subclavian venous thrombosis. This 28-year-old lady developed marked venous engorgement over the chest and neck. She was on the contraceptive pill. A venogram showed thrombosis of the subclavian vein. The patient improved after treatment with heparin but she did not return to normal completely. Surgical thrombectomy is rarely useful in such cases.

306

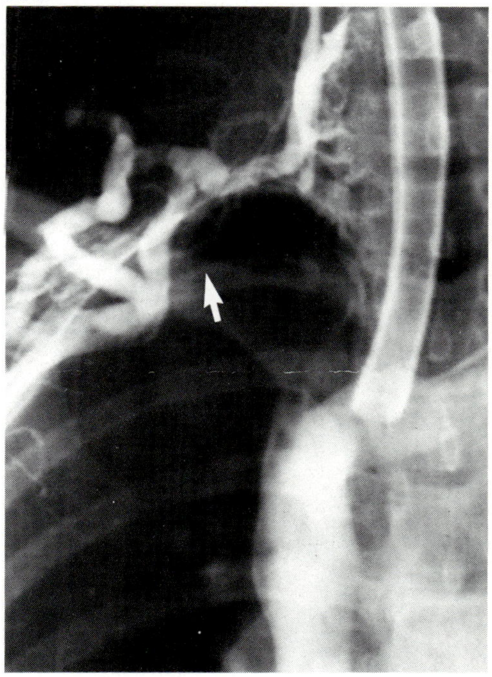

306 Subclavian venous blockage. Venography in the patient in **305** showed extensive blockage of the subclavian vein.

307

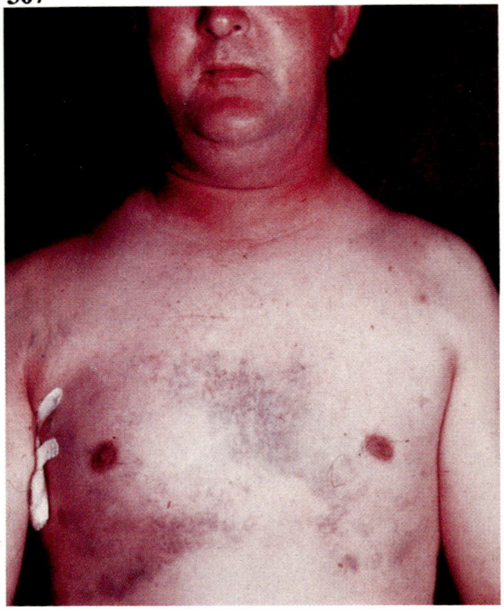

307 Occlusion of the superior vena cava is most commonly due to tumour round the vein causing compression. It produces bluish-red swollen appearance of upper chest and neck with prominent permanently filled veins.

308

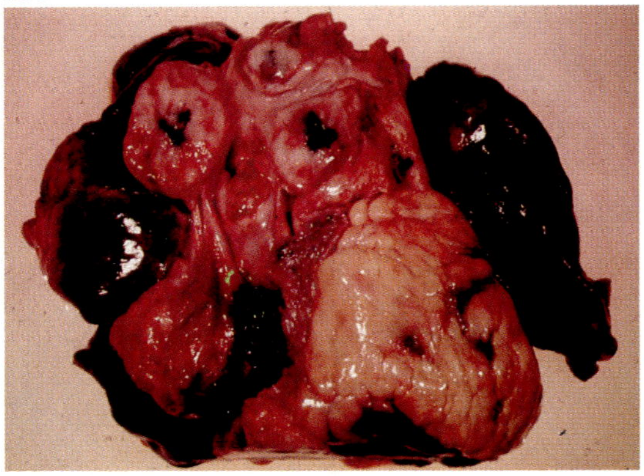

308 Vena cava clot. At post mortem malignant glands surrounded the upper end of the superior vena cava at the division. The opening of the subclavian vein can be seen. Clot is present in the lower part of the cava.

309

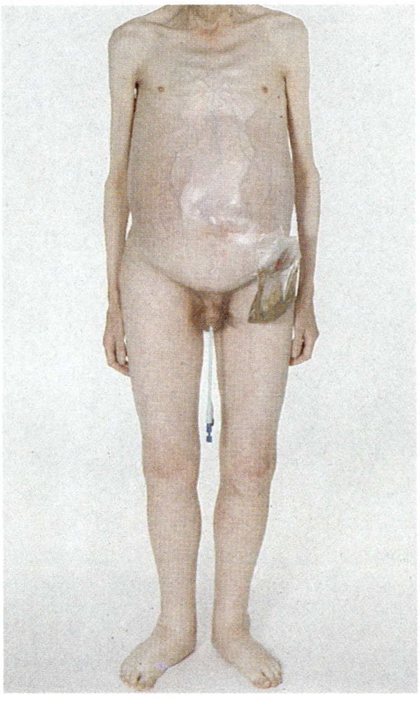

309 Inferior vena caval blockage is also associated with malignant disease as in this case. The distended veins in the abdomen and lower chest and oedema of the legs are noticeable.

310

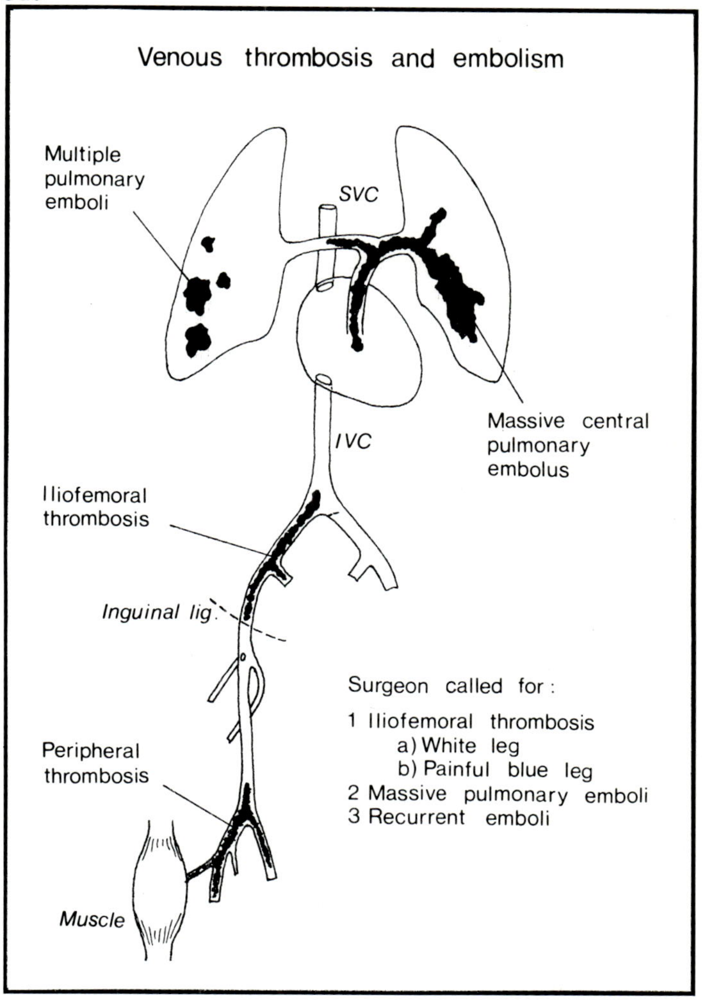

310 Thrombosis in the lower limb veins may lead to embolisation to the lungs. This diagram illustrates sites of venous thrombosis and types of pulmonary embolisms.

311

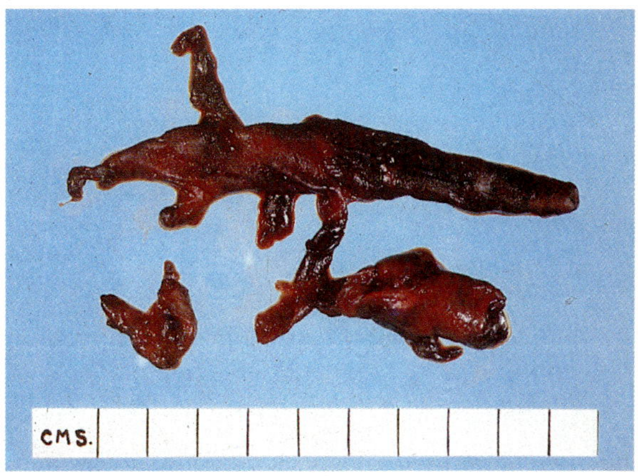

311 A pulmonary embolus may cause sudden death, rapid demise or recurrent chest pain and blood- stained sputum. This thrombus was removed from the pulmonary artery of a woman post-partum, by emergency Trendelenburg operation. Unfortunately the operation was carried out too late. Multiple small emboli with survival may lead to pulmonary hypertension.

11 Lymphatic system

Lymphoedema is classified into two main groups:

Primary lymphoedema

Congenital

Praecox i.e. appears early in life
Tarda i.e. appears after age of 35 years

Secondary lymphoedema

This is secondary to blockage or destruction of lymph nodes or channels from radiotherapy, malignant disease, surgery or tropical conditions.

312

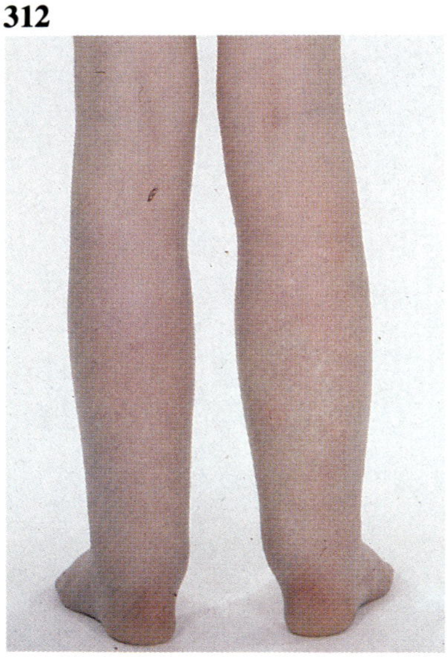

312 Primary lymphoedema in a boy of 15 years who had swollen legs from an early age, gradually getting worse. A strong family history was present (Milroy's disease).

313

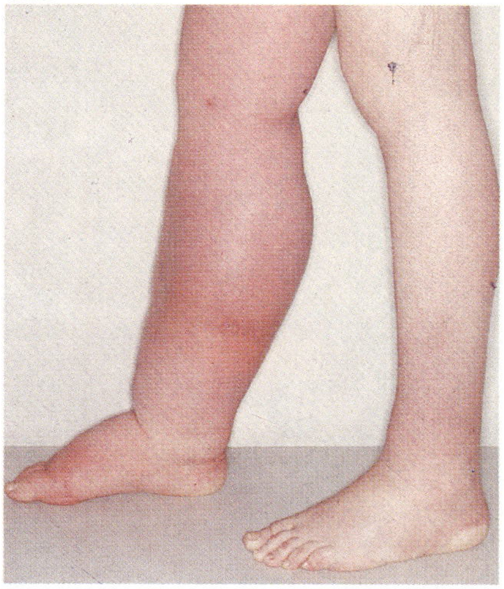

313 Primary lymphoedema in this case unilateral and may remain so or progress to become bilateral. The oedema is soft and easily pitted in the early stages but later pitting is absent or minimal.

314

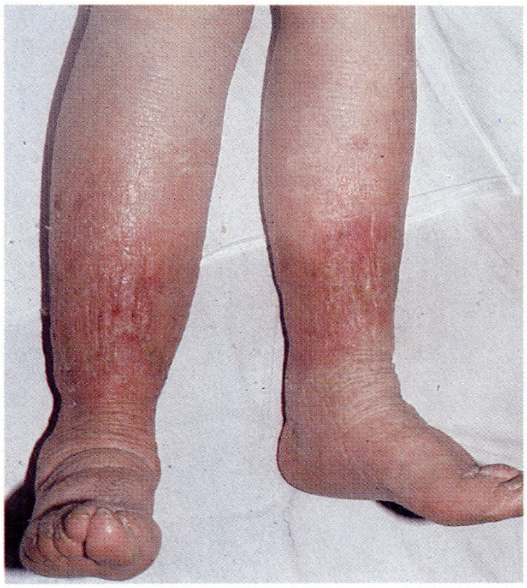

314 Primary lymphoedema (tarda). This appeared in a lady in her early forties. Now nearly 50 years, it is marked with presence of cellulitis which is recurrent and very troublesome.

315

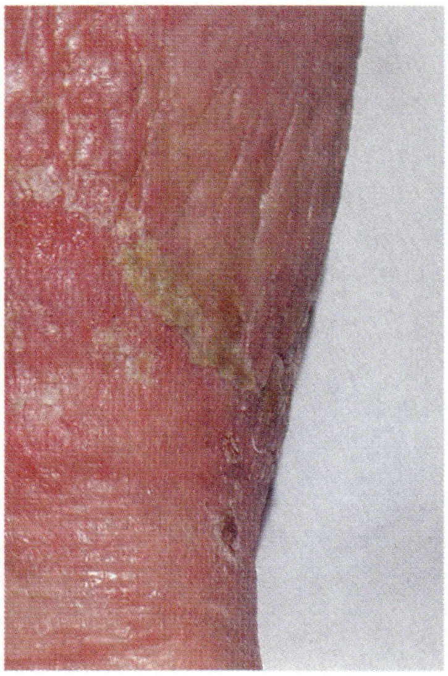

315 Primary lymphoedema. The close up in the above patient shows the thickening which can go on to an 'elephantiasis' like appearance.

316

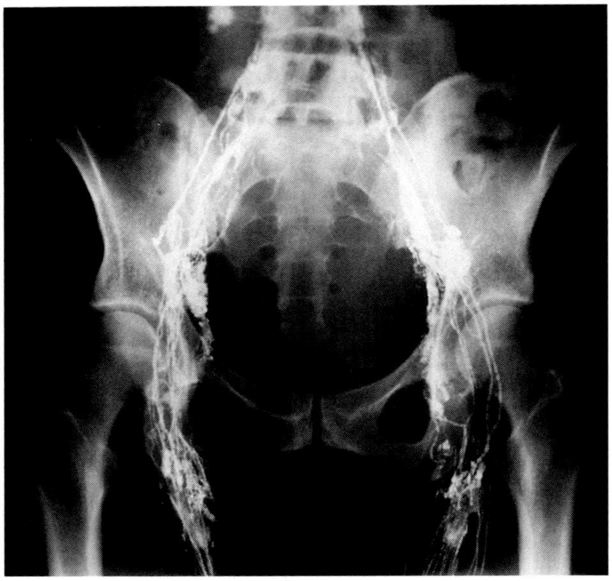

316 A normal lymphangiogram showing the upper end. The vessels are numerous and stream through the lymph nodes, which are normal in size.

317

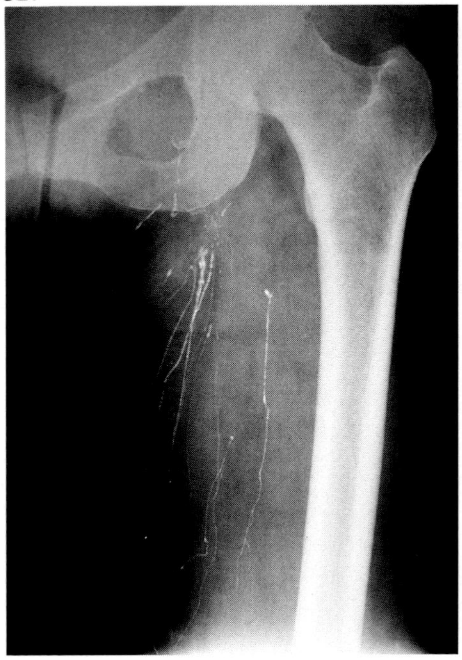

317 Hypoplasia. By contrast the lymphatic channels are spidery in appearance. In hypoplasia the vessels are fewer than normal and indeed may be difficult to find for cannulation.

318

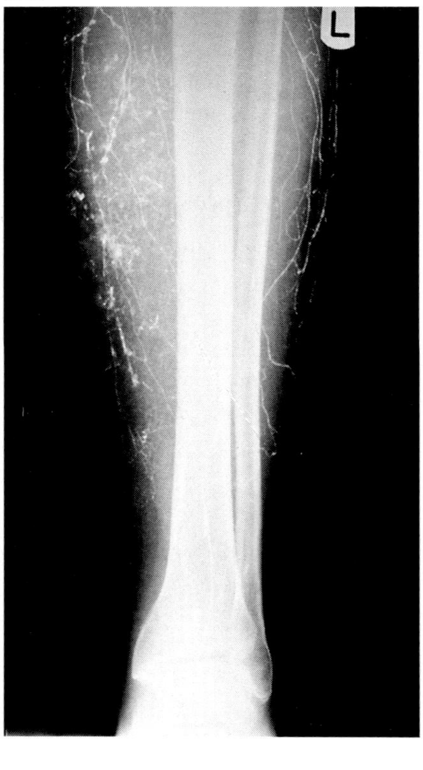

318 Lymphatic hyperplasia is less commonly found in lymphoedema, and is secondary to hypoplasia of the proximal lymphatics with obstruction to the lymph flow.

319

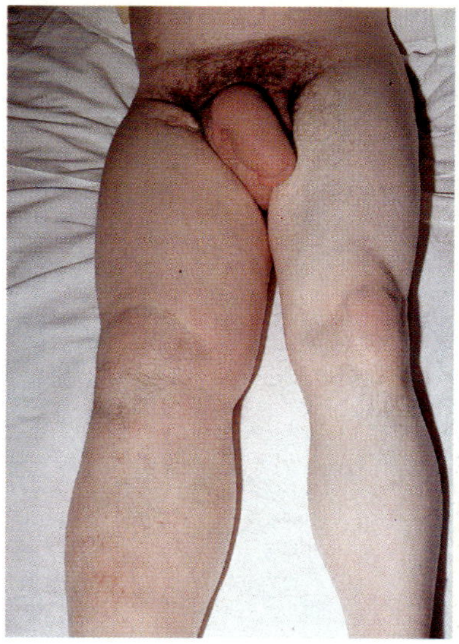

319 Secondary lymphoedema in this case was due to blockage by malignant disease affecting the glands in the groin. It can also follow blockage of lymphatics by radiation especially after radical mastectomy and also in a varicose ulcer; it can become extensive as a result of fibrosis.

Tumours of lymphatic vessels

320

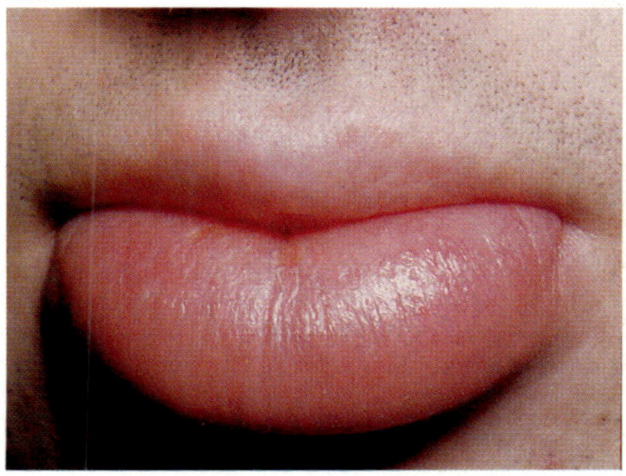

320 Macrocheilia. This lymphangioma has involved the lower lip producing a macrocheilia.

321

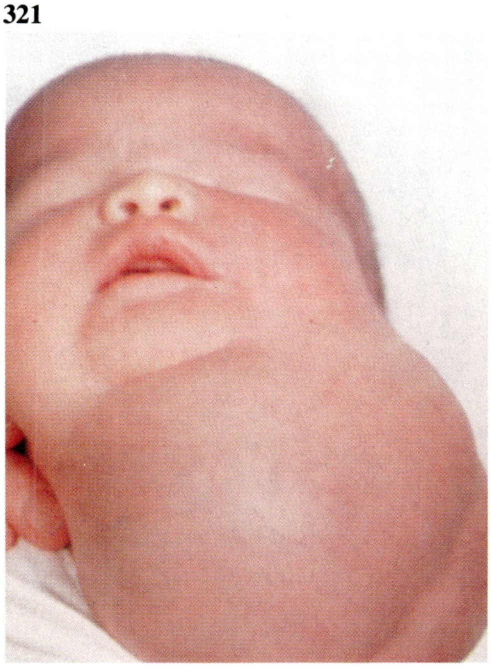

321 Cystic hygroma occurs most commonly in the neck, less so in the axilla. It is a multilocular cystic tumour which can be injected with sclerosants or excised. In this baby the swelling completely disappeared within two years without treatment.

322

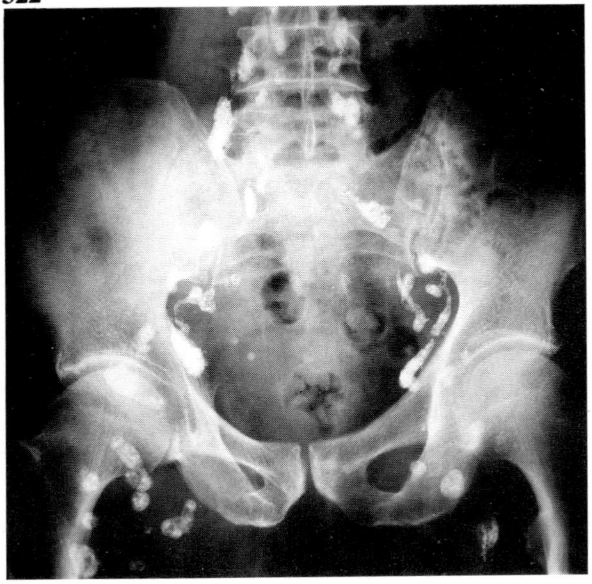

322 Hodgkin's disease may cause extensive involvement of the inguinal, iliac and abdominal glands, as shown here in a 50-year-old patient.

323

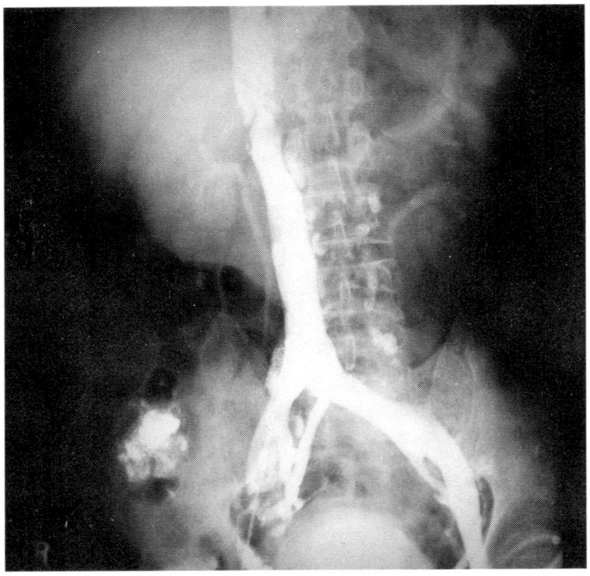

323 The nodes in Hodgkin's disease may be large enough to indent the inferior vena cava, as shown in this combined lymphangiogram and venogram.

Index

B

C

D

E

F

G

H

I

K

L

M

N

O

P

U

V

W

X